3,000
PULSES

Surviving Depression with TMS
Transcranial Magnetic Stimulation

A MEMOIR

Martha Rhodes

with -

Randy Ian Pardell, MD DFAPA

I AM I BOOKS
Hyde Park, NY

Published by I Am I Books, Inc.
370 Violet Avenue
Poughkeepsie, NY 12601
www.iamibooks.com

Copyright ©2012 by Martha Rhodes

First Edition 2012

Author's Note: The events described in this memoir are true. Some names
have been replaced by pseudonyms in order to protect privacy, particularly
those of medical personnel.

This book is intended to reflect the life experiences of the author and in no
way should it be considered to be medical advice, recommendations for
treatment, or a replacement for medical care given by physicians or trained
medical personnel.

Printed in the United States of America.

Cover design by Robert Guy and Nicole Lalama.

Cover photo obtained from www.iStockphoto.com.

Back cover photography by Steven Robinson.

ISBN: 978-0-9855339-0-8

Distributed by I Am I Books, Inc.
370 Violet Avenue
Poughkeepsie, NY 12601
www.iamibooks.com

For John

"Everyone should have a love like this."

3,000
PULSES

Surviving Depression with TMS
Transcranial Magnetic Stimulation

A Memoir

Contents

As a clinical psychiatrist for more than twenty years, I started performing Transcranial Magnetic Stimulation on my patients in December, 2009 at my Poughkeepsie, New York office. My patients who suffered severe depression and who had not responded to medication or psychotherapeutic treatment were experiencing extremely positive results with TMS. My desire to write about such a groundbreaking technology and the impressive results of its therapeutic power became a reality when I met Martha Rhodes one year later.

Martha had started writing a book about her long history of depression, her suicide attempt and multiple treatment failures, and ultimately finding life-saving relief with TMS. She knew she needed a medical consultant to advise her. I wanted to write about the hope Transcranial Magnetic Stimulation treatment offered, and I welcomed the idea of collaborating on a book project to spread the word about this new breakthrough in the treatment of severe depression. A TMS Therapy Consultant, Joy Patermo, knew of both our efforts and fortuitously arranged a meeting for us.

In February 2011 we met at an Italian restaurant. Martha greeted me with a warm and engaging smile—her typical approach those days. During the next two hours over hearty bowls of pasta, Martha described her insidious descent into persistent depression punctuated by weight gain and emotional numbing with antidepressant side effects. I have used medications to treat psychiatric conditions throughout my entire career and I am aware of the potential side effects she experienced. However, Martha's dramatic portrayals of her spiral into alcohol use to self-medicate her depression, her suicide attempt, and subsequent hospitalizations moved me.

Psychiatrists often become inured to the depths of our patients' emotional pain, but Martha's openness and honesty broke through any wall I had built. I was startled and dismayed by her inpatient hospital experience. I experienced frustration as I learned of her failed medication trials after her hospitalization and worsening side effects, as well as her withdrawal symptoms from abrupt discontinuation of the drugs. Martha's story graphically describes her quest to find her way out of a severe depression that nearly took her life.

It is often a quantum leap for psychiatrists to recommend new treatments that are not well known, unless a pharmaceutical representative details the science to a physician, or the science is discussed at an attended professional meeting. Martha met up with this resistance as her psychiatrists and insurance company did not recommend or provide coverage for her TMS therapy. They encouraged her to either undergo Electroconvulsive Therapy, a more expensive treatment with a worse side-effect burden of memory loss, or to continue with futile medication trials with significant, deleterious side effects.

Martha described her trepidation about her lack of an initial response during the early stage of her TMS treatment, but eventually she had an unmistakable lifting of her depression. She has remained in remission of her depression symptoms since that time.

From our first meeting, Martha and I have forged a deep and abiding friendship and collaborative relationship. We have initiated one of the first TMS monthly support groups in the nation. We have spread the message about TMS therapy as a highly effective vehicle on the path for depression recovery when medications don't work. We have lectured throughout the Northern U.S. about the power of TMS therapy and how patients with depression are showing awakening responses. We encourage physicians and mental health clinicians to refer patients who are in need of an alternative and provide them with ongoing support during their TMS process.

Recently I attended a conference at Beth Israel-Deaconess Hospital hosted by Harvard Medical School and the Berenson-Allen Center for Noninvasive Brain Stimulation. I asked Dr. Alvaro Pascual-Leone, one of the world's leading experts on TMS, what he believes the impact of TMS therapy will be for the future of psychiatry. He stated clearly, "TMS will have a transformational impact on psychiatry." It is my experience that our patients are having that "transformational" awakening from their depression. TMS alleviates the painful symptoms of the depressive brain disease—but in a manner that is muted not by antidepressant side effects, but rather with a clarity and vitality that I have not see in my entire psychiatric career.

I am grateful to Martha for sharing her life experience with me as she has humanized the clinical syndrome of depression. Her story is one of redemption. It is an indictment of our profession of psychiatry and the medical insurance industry, but also illustrative of the power of medical science to ameliorate the devastating brain disease of depression.

I hope that in reading Martha's story and the hard-won but successful results she has achieved, you will find a new and exciting option for resolving depression in you or your loved ones. TMS treatment centers are opening in all parts of the United States, and the promise of help for the hopeless shines ever brighter.

Randy Ian Pardell, MD DFAPA
July 2012

It was the easiest decision I ever made. Easier than choosing a nail polish color. Like rolling off a log. A simple cry of "Uncle" and it's done. Pour the vodka, open the amber bottle, and fill the left hand with the thirty little white pills. Open the mouth, shove them all in, and send them on their way down the gullet with the potent liquid. No thoughts. No worries. Feeling absolutely nothing.

Done, done, and done.

Although I took antidepressants religiously and repeatedly conferred with my doctors as to their declining effect, psychotropic medications have taken me down an untenable path of confusion and failure—one that has driven me to examine where I went on February 25, 2009. That's the date I downed an entire bottle of Xanax, not without the help of excessive pours of wine and vodka, and all with the hope of ending what appeared to be a perfect life.

Twenty years earlier …

I wait alone on the dark corner of Seventy-Ninth Street and Amsterdam Avenue in New York City. I nudge my coat's collar to my cheeks, wondering if the cross-town bus will arrive before the cold, March wind proves it the loser in the battle to keep me warm. A mental switch flips itself on, and suddenly I viscerally experience myself standing next to myself, feeling at once the actor and an audience member in the same movie. As the bus approaches, I envision meeting its front end head-on with a full body block. I stand frozen in my own private scene: the performer waiting for my cue to jump—the observer wondering if I actually will.

I cut to reality. The bus door flips open. In robotic motion, I ascend the steps, deposit the fare, and drop my heavy body into the nearest empty seat. We head across Central Park toward a friend's apartment where I will spend the night alone, minding her cat.

That was the early 1990s. Despite my rising career in New York City advertising at that time, I had been sinking into an emotional pit for several years as I simultaneously worked a full-time job and raised our two young children with my husband, John. The frighteningly real bus stop fantasy, and the palpable feelings behind it, haunted me for weeks. A group of supportive friends with whom I shared the troubling scenario suggested I seek the help of a psychiatrist, who in turn diagnosed me with clinical depression and recommended an antidepressant medication. The subsequent first prescription of Zoloft aided and abetted my ability to regain a mental footing and fortified an emotional façade from my early forties throughout the following two decades.

Although I was glad to have relief from the strain of trying to keep it all together, the drug prescribed for me presented side effects that at the time seemed a small price to pay for my loftier goal of being alright in the eyes of the world. Initially, it warded off any despairing thoughts and laid an armored cloak over my hopelessness, replacing it with a comfortable, impenetrable numbness. I became lulled into a false sense of being cured by the drug, fostered by an uninformed belief that all I had to do to sustain my mental health was remember to take the prescribed daily happy pill.

I grew from a sassy Size 8 to an unrecognizable Size 16— one of the medication's many side effects. That fact only served to exacerbate my depression, lowering my self-esteem and obliterating any desire to maintain sexual intimacy in my marriage. The day I found myself relegated to the Women's clothing racks, shuffling through sizes 1X, 2X, and 3X, only confirmed that I was no longer the former Miss Connecticut beauty pageant contestant with all the tricks of the beauty trade in my svelte hip pocket. I viewed the person in the dressing room mirror as a total stranger, disgusted with what peered back at me, longing for my former self, yet knowing in my heart she was gone forever. "Is this what happens when the girl becomes the woman?" I disdainfully asked myself. "Are we expected to leave our pretty selves behind in order to move forward in the process of living?"

With the added physical girth and lonely detachment from a healthy marital relationship, my energy and lust for life waned proportionately. Nothing made sense to me—not physically, mentally, or emotionally. Life's ultimatums boiled down to this: if I didn't take the antidepressant medication, I would not be able to hold down a job. I would fail my children and lose my marriage. I would not survive. Heavy body, heavy thoughts, heavy heart.

Had I been warned of the drug's hideous side effects, I might have chosen to not take it, but on the other hand I really had no choice. By the time I awoke to the fact that Zoloft made me fat, I also knew it kept me on an even keel and I was too scared to try to live without it. My Catholic mother's classic recommendation for any of life's difficulties resurfaced: "Just offer it up for the souls in Purgatory, Martha." I wondered if the souls in Purgatory felt as depressed as I did on Earth, and if they'd ever pray for me if the shoe were on the other foot. Nevertheless, tolerating several other antidepressants' side effects became my own personal cross to bear. The numbness the medications induced served to replace any normal emotions, making it easier to cope with life's problems, but in the bargain they left me passionless. Eventually the drugs became ineffective, and unbeknownst to my primary care physician and myself, I tumbled down the treacherous rabbit hole.

The reality of my attempted suicide will never elude me. I live a guarded existence fully aware of how easy it was to step over life's edge. I continue to ask myself the obvious, unrelenting questions that demand answers in order for me to go on living. How did I, a successful, ostensibly stable person, get so far away from a good life? Where did I go that February night in 2009? How did I even get there? How could I find my way back? Would I ever really get back to where I was—and did I even want to rejoin that place? And most important, because of my history with depression and how antidepressants affected me, was I ever really here in the first place?

1 | ANATOMY OF A BREAK-APART

"Life is real! Life is earnest! And the grave is not its goal…"

— Henry Wadsworth Longfellow, *The Psalm of Life*

My earliest memories are infused with an ever-nagging sadness that underscored even the happiest days of my life. Childhood experiences were eclipsed by sad, nervous feelings that infiltrated my teenage and adult years. The subject of death and dying automatically evoked a certain cavalier yet unspoken attitude in me. I didn't fear death one bit. My fascination with how I would actually like to "go" kept me preoccupied throughout the years—a car crash, a sudden heart attack, a slow-simmering cancer. I also spent an inordinate amount of time contemplating what is on the other side: Heaven, Hell, Purgatory, reincarnation, or perhaps nothingness. Although my father's sudden death initially shattered my heart, I ultimately felt a private sense of jealousy. *Now he's got the real picture. Now he knows what's really going on here and there.* I also envied my dad for getting out early. He spent his fifty-eighth birthday on his deathbed.

Living a long life never appealed to me. It always looked like too much work to get through an imagined day at the age of, say, ninety-six. Whenever I'd see an ancient soul struggle to cross the street, push a grocery cart, or bring a quivering fork to her mouth in a restaurant, I'd declare under my breath, "Just shoot me!" I threw an over-the-top fiftieth birthday party for myself, replete with beachside lobster bake, live jazz music, antique merry-go-round. To everyone's delight, a rare, full-spectrum rainbow from a spontaneous rain shower heralded a brilliant sunset on Long

Island Sound. I guess I figured I might as well throw the big one at fifty since I believed I'd be gone by my sixtieth.

As the years wore on well past that fiftieth birthday, I habitually greeted each day with a palpable ennui, sometimes bordering on dread. "Okay, Martha, you can make yourself do this!" I coaxed myself, as I moved into an unconscious, bored, automaton state: brushing teeth, showering, dressing, getting out the door, and then donning my game face (read: big smile, congenial attitude, pour on the enthusiasm). The truth is, it got me places.

How I ended up in the corner office of more than one major New York advertising agency remains a mystery to me. Vice President, Senior VP, Managing Partner. I tried to make it seem very easy for me, all the while impressing family and friends. I delighted in the idea that I could pull off such a career charade. Unfortunately, maintaining my game face while struggling through chronic depression eventually levied a heavy toll on my body and soul.

Don't misunderstand. I wanted those positions. I aspired to be the best I could be in every job challenge handed to me. I regarded my monthly Metro North train pass for the two-and-a-half-hour commute as a badge of courage. Earning a six-figure salary equaled the proverbial brass ring. At times I felt secretly guilty for accepting the sympathy of others for what they perceived as superhuman career efforts.

"Oh, Martha, you work twelve-hour days in New York and then do a two-and-a-half-hour commute to get home and make dinner for John and the kids? How do you do it?" They weren't exactly wrong—it was a difficult lifestyle, with two small children, a husband, and a house to run. Nevertheless, I had my groove going with no desire to change anything. Even when my jobs were lost due to layoffs, changes in upper management, and justified resignations, my fertile network of colleagues and contacts moved me into the next job like a duck on water—and always accompanied by a bigger title and higher salary.

What more could a person ask for?

At one point a close friend offered to sublet her studio apartment to me so I could live in the city during the week, thereby eliminating the arduous race for trains morning and evening. The free time reclaimed in the bargain were an added bonus. I soon found myself working longer days and keeping after work dates for drinks and dinners with friends thanks to those available hours. I had the best of both worlds, or so I thought, living in a trendy New York neighborhood by myself Monday through Thursday, returning Friday night to the cozy existence with my husband of thirty-plus years in our quaint suburban home. Since we were empty nesters by that time, the phrase "absence makes the heart grow fonder" neatly applied. Again, what more could a person ask for?

I suppose that "what" should have been a clearer perspective regarding my psychological health. I had no awareness of the price tag attached to this best-of-both-worlds arrangement. For someone as buttoned up as I considered myself to be—running multilevel departments of employees, meeting impossible deadlines, and managing million-dollar-plus budgets—I spent many of those solitary evenings in the apartment consumed with self-doubt, loneliness, and feelings of intense futility. Balancing a career, spending so much time alone without my husband, and relying solely on an ineffective antidepressant to smooth my rough emotional edges proved to be an unsuccessful formula for my life. Most medical professionals would call my condition severe clinical depression, and my depression had moved in as an unannounced roommate.

The insanity of petty advertising account executives, the frustrations of misunderstood art directors, the endless concern for racking up billable hours to clients who chronically increased their expectations while reducing their already shallow budgets— it all reeked of senseless expenditure of my energy, save for that big, fat bimonthly paycheck. "What's the point of any of this?"

I constantly muttered. The muttering's volume soon increased to an internal wail, audible only to myself. In retrospect, I realized I equated my sense of worth with my basic job identity and my ability to make money—nothing more, and certainly nothing less.

Oblivious to the looming collision course my behavior charted during those years, I stuck to my motto: Just proceed. It's what kept me on the Employee A-list in the business world. "Give the problem to Martha. She'll get it done. She's the one who can figure it out!"

The tenets for my life started with being trusted and dependable. Do not disappoint friends, no matter what. But those same good friends, had they known what price I paid for that commitment, would certainly have dissuaded me, never allowing what turned out to be a codependent behavior pattern. What I presumed to be a positive attribute was actually an intense need to control any and all situations. It's the old Irving Berlin song from *Annie Get Your Gun*: "Anything You Can Do I Can Do Better." The more I could control and succeed, the less depressed I unconsciously imagined I would feel. The control and busy-ness kept me out of the depression cave. Whenever sad and hopeless feelings crept in, the busier I became—a vicious survival cycle.

As a middle child in a gaggle of seven, one who was highly excitable and hypersensitive to life in general, I recognized at an early age that my frequent temper tantrums not only drained me physically, they got me into big trouble with the grown-ups. In self-defense I developed the habit of rarely shedding a tear, even where it would have been appropriate. I remember touting such a success to my father: "I didn't cry even once today, Daddy!" I actually considered this an accomplishment at the tender age of five or six. Sucking it up and proving to myself and everyone else just what a together kind of gal I could be, I maintained this stoic, can-do attitude throughout my teens and into adulthood—until my resistance to life's pain began to wear thin.

A pervasive melancholy had underpinned my mood for several

weeks prior to the fateful night I called it quits. I impetuously responded to the mental goading of "I'm done! Take this job, er, life, and shove it!" that evening. I had expressed it to my sister a few weeks earlier as, "I feel really sad lately. And whenever I see, hear, smell anything, I'm reminded only of the past, with no sense at all of the future." At the time it seemed like an innocuous observation for both of us. But the evening I overdosed, alone with my thoughts and emotions, a tsunami of futility and despair crashed onto my emotional shores.

I had been out to dinner with some business associates. When I returned to the apartment later that evening, I made the mistake of checking work-related E-mail. Upper management change was in motion, and everyone felt its pressure. Suddenly the desperate, reactive content of the crisscrossing E-mails struck me as so absurd—so futile—that I lost all logic and desire to respond to them. The issue of change at work was not the real issue, however. I had been through management shifts in other agencies—it was the nature of the advertising business. But because depression was eroding my ability to cope with life in general, and the antidepressant medication I took every morning had lost its efficacy, this particular situation simply became a very deadly catalyst to let myself off of life's hook.

Irrational musings began chattering in my mind: Nicholas and Elizabeth were grown adults now, leading successful lives of their own—*they don't need me now.* (I already felt I only deserved a C+ grade as a mom.) *They'd be better off without me anyway.* As for growing old with my husband—*He'll have an easier time of it without me—I'm just a depressed load of a temperamental wife who'll never be happy, no matter what.*

A distinct calmness settled in and around me. I ceased thinking about anything or anyone. My mind and body felt so intensely exhausted that even going to sleep seemed like too much effort. I simply did not want to live another day. The previous months' grumblings of how feebly my life measured up to life's randomness and how pointless everything in it really was climaxed to a crescendo I'd never heard before.

I poured myself a glass of straight Stolichnaya vodka on the rocks and began the descent into the final dark abyss. I found the full bottle of Xanax I kept for emergency anxiety attacks but had never used for fear of their addictive reputation. I became very still, very calm. Time and place magically evaporated.

In three words: I gave up.

∾

Although my brother Michael and I didn't have a close relationship per se and I didn't have his phone number conveniently in my phone contacts, I was later told that I called him to "say goodbye." I have no recollection of this, but perhaps I chose to call him rather than any of my other six siblings because I'd known for some time that Michael battled his own lifetime demons. Maybe I felt he would be the one to truly understand what it meant to be so depressed, so hopeless, so exhausted from life. Perhaps telling him I was ending my own life would somehow afford me permission and understanding from our brothers and sisters. Or maybe a long lost spirit deep inside me really did want to live, and perhaps he would sound the alarm. To this day I do not know the answer.

I asked him not to tell anyone but, I am told, Michael contacted one sister who knew the street address who told another sister who lived closest to the city who called 911, whose emergency services responders then had to go through the neighboring apartment at midnight and break through the back door to haul me away on a stretcher to the nearest emergency room. Everyone got in on the act of my very implausible drama. I guess being one of seven children proved to be a true blessing this time.

The next stop on my life's commuter train—Saint Vincent's Hospital emergency room, gallantly escorted by New York's finest, the FDNY's EMT brigade. Two days later I finally woke up with a round-the-clock guard at my bedside, who disallowed even a trip to the toilet without her watchful eye. I naively regarded this as the hospital's routine policy of excellent patient care, which it was. However, it didn't take me long to see it more accurately as someone guarding a psycho patient who just might make a second, more successful attempt at her own demise. This is when I had the rudest awakening of my life thus far. I suddenly realized I had put myself in the uncharted waters of the mental health care system—and little did I know of the shocking consequences awaiting me in the coming weeks.

Curious people often ask a person who has survived a suicide attempt why he or she did it and what they felt when they realized they didn't die. For myself, I felt absolutely nothing. Neither worried nor relieved; not happy, not sad; not angry or disappointed; simply numb, vacant of any sense of past, present, and future. To the question "Why?" I had no answer either. To this day, all I know is that it was as easy as anything I'd ever done in my life—seamless, swift, and random. No planning, no thinking, no feeling. Repercussions affecting my family and friends were absent from the equation. The event was peaceful, personal, quiet.

Not until my family showed up around my hospital bed revealing no signs of anger, judgment, or shock did I begin to catch a glimmer of my life's true meaning. What I saw was unconditional love, concern, encouragement, and kindness. That's when I began to regret my actions, to finally feel the pain.

And most important, I cried.

2 | Wake-up Call

"She's thirsty—can't we give her something to drink?"
I remember… my six-foot-four son Nicholas's anxious voice wafting
above my head, his enormous fingers struggling to slip ice chips into
my mouth like a mother bird feeding her chick; my sister Nicole's
gentle hands on my foot, massaging it with reassuring care as she
cooed hope into the emergency room's flustered atmosphere.
"You're gonna be okay, Martha, you're going to make it."
I slipped back into unconsciousness.

The winter sun shining through my hospital room window beckoned me back to reality. So did the large, starkly bright room, the smell of clean linens enveloping my exhausted body, distant murmurs of nurses and aides in the hallway, and my mouth so dry I could hardly feel my tongue. My consciousness begged to have this be a dream as I slowly grasped what had become of me since the night before in the apartment. There was no denying the reality of this situation—I had stepped over a forbidden line into a world I had always feared, with nobody to blame but myself.

John stood by my bedside—the good husband, stunned as anyone could be—mercifully withholding the judgment a less benevolent man would no doubt dish out. His warm, familiar hand in mine felt like my soul's only lifeline, although the IVs, Foley catheter, and oxygen tube dutifully supported my bodily functions as I drifted in and out of awareness.

I had never been a fan of hospitals for a myriad of reasons, the main one being my aversion to the physical and emotional vulnerability that accompanies hospital confinement. When I was in my late twenties, I spent six weeks at my father's bedside while he succumbed to cancer. The profound emotional experience of shepherding him to the other side left me believing hospitals were meant for dying. When I became pregnant with our children years later, I chose to deliver them both at home with a very caring, competent doctor, along with my willing husband and some of my siblings in attendance.

A few years after the home birth experiences, an unavoidable week-long hospital stay due to an extreme case of pneumonia served to reinforce this loathing. An abusive eleven-to-seven night shift aide thunderously berated my elderly hospital roommate every night for a variety of geriatric mishaps beyond this poor patient's control. Unable to clearly see the aide in the dark room, in my mind's eye her deep voice alone portrayed her as an oversized Amazon as her heavy steps slapped the linoleum floor.

"You pressed the buzzer 'cause you said you needed the bedpan, you stupid woman! So what's it this time—another false alarm? How many times do I have to go through this with you tonight, huh?"

The attendant's rage mushroomed as she flung the empty bedpan into the bed stand with such force it clanged loudly enough to wake someone in a coma. I wanted to get a good look at her so I would know to avoid her in the future, but instead I hid my head under the covers for fear she would see me awake and manufacture a reason to come after me. The concept of playing possum in a hospital seemed incongruous.

Shortly after my release I received a patient satisfaction survey in the mail from the hospital. My pneumonia had been successfully treated but the trauma of those few nights of anxiousness and fear had not healed. Indignation set in. In the "Comments" section on the form, I described the situation and my reaction to it. Within days of returning the survey someone from the hospital's Human Relations Department called me on the telephone for further clarification as to what had happened.

"Look, I'm not trying to get anyone fired from her job," I cautioned, "but the nurse's aide who treated that poor old lady next to me so badly shouldn't have any patient contact. Put her in the laundry room or the hospital kitchen, but get her off the floor. She has anger issues and she's in the wrong job."

When I hung up the phone that day, the vulnerability I felt while lying in that hospital bed came rushing back to me. I realized how humiliating a bedpan is and how not being permitted to shower and wash my hair only made me feel sicker. I resented that my children weren't allowed to visit me. The constant interruptions for temperature, medications, and blood pressure checks left me feeling like a powerless, sick prisoner. I vowed that in the future I would avoid hospitals at all costs.

Thirty years later, I wished I had remembered that old promise when I took the pills in the apartment that fateful night or had at least imagined that a failed suicide attempt could lead to hospitalization. Perhaps I might have given self-destruction a second thought or tried a more effective way to do it.

No one could have been more surprised than I, therefore, to find myself lying in a bed that first morning in Saint Vincent's Hospital in New York City.

By the second day the routine clatter of hospital activity in the corridor finally brought me out of my stupor.

John must have gone home to Connecticut, I thought to myself as I eyed the breakfast tray perched on my bed table. *I didn't even hear them bring it in—I was so sound asleep. It must be cold by now. Otherwise I'd smell something warm, wouldn't I?*

I rolled over and closed my eyes again, struggling to think clearly and trying to grasp what had happened to me, but perfectly willing to tread water rather than swim out of the deep end. I didn't have the strength or desire to imagine the future—it felt too scary and took way too much energy.

My retreat into suspended reality was short-lived. By mid-morning I discovered I was fair game for a gang of psychiatry interns making rounds in search of the quintessential case by which to hone their newly acquired medical skills. I'm sure it's not every day a failed suicide attempt shows up, so my arrival must have made their day.

I re-awoke to an audience of several furrow-browed novices appropriately clad in crisp, white lab coats, studiously staring at me as I tried to answer their teacher's rapid-fire questions.

"Mrs. Rhodes, do you know where you are? Do you remember what happened to you? Do you know what you did? Can you tell us how you are feeling? Are you hearing any strange voices? Do you think you will try to harm yourself again?" His voice leaked a distinct tone of admonishment. He clung to his clipboard and peered at me over the top of his eyeglasses (when he even bothered to look at me at all). I felt like a repentant, scolded child anticipating a spanking.

A soupy fog shrouded my mind as I blurted out whatever answers seemed acceptable.

"Yes, I'm in the hospital." "No, well, I don't remember much." "I do remember what I did." "I think I feel okay, just very tired." "No, no strange voices." "I don't know if I can answer that, 'if I'll harm myself again.' I don't think so, but I'm just too tired."

I couldn't think straight. Not only could I not focus my thoughts, I felt exhausted, alone, and scared beyond description. In a normal situation I would have asked, "Who are you? Why are there so many of you standing there? Why do you need to know this information? What are you intending to do with it? May I have a moment to think about these things, please?"

Clearly this interrogation put me on an uneven playing field. I didn't have John by my side, and my usual analytical mind and keen intuition had vanished. As the interns traipsed out of the room they left me with a confused, befuddled feeling that hinted of trouble down the road. I wept, lonely and afraid, knowing I desperately needed someone to help me navigate this foreign territory.

In the afternoon lull following the morning's flurry of hospital procedures—noisy breakfast carts, doctors' rounds, nurses checking vitals, linen changes, and sundry other necessities—I rested quietly in a guarded limbo with intermittent naps. The voices of two excited but hushed female voices stirred me awake in the late afternoon.

"Oh, look, Coraline, honey—they gave you the bed right next to a nice big sunny winda." My new roommate arrived on a gurney accompanied by a tall, elegantly dressed woman who sidled alongside her like an anxious tour guide. Her authoritative carriage matched her clear, sonorous voice. She rolled a well-traveled suitcase and two shopping bags overflowing with stuffed animals and fluffy slippers. One strap of an oversized, multicolored cloth bag hung on to her shoulder for dear life as she maneuvered her large frame between the end of my bed and the stretcher. Another even more demonstrative voice trailed in through the door behind them.

"Oh, how luvly, sista. This is the finest room you've been in since we got to New York City. This is just fahn, very fahn." I instantly detected her strong southern accent when she leaned so heavily on the word "fine." She wore a deep violet felt hat with a sweeping brim that curiously hid half her face. Although I couldn't see her, I felt her positive loving energy as she and her other sister fussed over their frail patient while the orderly gently coaxed her onto the bed next to mine.

As soon as Coraline settled in, the two sisters dutifully went about adjusting the curtains, pouring her water, fluffing her pillow, and positioning several personal items on her bed stand. Only then did they notice my fascinated stare.

"Oh, my, have we disturbed you, ma'am? We are so sorry to be makin' such a fuss, but we're here to take care of our sista who's fixin' to have a special surgery in a day or two. Now, can we get you anythin' for yo' self while we're at it?"

I quickly averted my eyes so as not to appear too nosey, not to mention the fact that I hardly felt in the mood for conversation.

"Uh, no, I'm fine. Very fine. Thank you, though."

They continued their sisterly chatter and I picked up on the fact that the third sister, my roommate, Coraline, was scheduled for a special procedure for a recurring cancer. They had converged in New York City from Washington, DC, South Carolina, and Mississippi with high hopes of joining forces to help Coraline win her battle.

I thought of my own three sisters and the many challenging times we shared, laughing and crying with each other over life's events. I envied Coraline, happy she had the comfort of her sisters and sad that I had almost removed myself from my own with my senseless act of attempted suicide. I had shared none of my desperation with any of my sisters prior to the night I collapsed. I had kept my death wish handily under wraps where nobody close to me could have even a hint of how low I truly felt.

I wondered what my family thought of me, now that I had unsuccessfully tried to vacate my position as the sister who could do anything and everything for them—the sister who always knew how to make things happen, figure out the problem, and get the job done; the sister with the sometimes uncomfortably strong personality and the mercurial emotions to go along with it. I wondered if they were as shocked as I was about what I'd done, or if they'd seen this disaster coming but feared holding up a "dangerous curve ahead" sign. I felt as if I'd failed everyone in my family, certain that my disdain for myself rivaled their disappointment in me.

∾

Other than a slight swoosh of air, the door barely made a sound as it swung into my hospital room. I almost didn't recognize the face hidden behind the thick woolen scarf protecting her rosy cheeks from the bitter New York winter.

My swollen, tearful eyes connected with my daughter Elizabeth's gorgeous smile as she wordlessly slipped through the doorway and into my arms. No one told me she was coming up from Florida. I would never have expected her to make such a long and sudden trip for me, but I could not have been happier to have her by my side at that moment.

After she graduated from college, Elizabeth had decided to leave her dancing and personal fitness career in the New York area and move to Miami, where she became a member of the Miami Beach Ocean Rescue team. The roots she set down in South Beach took, and we only saw her twice a year at best. It was difficult having my only daughter live so far away and even harder to have her show up in this disastrous circumstance.

"Mommeeeee ... how are you feeling?" I could feel the winter coldness on her cheek as she pressed a kiss onto mine. The smell of the outside world clung to her jacket even as she tossed it on the chair next to my bed.

"I didn't know you were coming—no one told me."

"I know. I wanted to surprise you. I asked Daddy not to say a word."

"I'm so grateful you're here, honey, thank you so much for coming," was all I could utter as I fumbled for more tissues, already trying to spare her emotions that couldn't have been more obvious.

"I'm so sorry it took me so long to get here. I couldn't get a flight, but I explained what happened and the airline agent helped get me a seat early this morning. I'm going to stay at your apartment so I'll be nearby and I can bring you anything you need."

As grateful as I felt to have my daughter at my side, eager to do whatever she could to help me, a twinge of guilt crept over me as I recognized I was no longer her all-knowing, strong mother. She was no longer my dependent little girl. Our roles had reversed themselves all too quickly, dramatically, and unexpectedly. "Thank you, honey. Thank you. I'm sorry. I'm just so very sorry for all of this."

She gave no reply. She climbed up on the bed next to me as her loving arm cradled my shoulders.

From infancy Elizabeth had always been a snuggle bug—comfortable in her own skin and generous with hugs, kisses, foot rubs, and warm affection. Never had I been more in need of these gifts than that day. We spent the rest of the afternoon chatting about her job of pulling overconfident, inept swimmers out of the ocean, her new personal training clients, and how different the climate is between Florida and New York. We were in the midst of one of the worst winters on record and that week happened to be the coldest of the year so far. At least my maternal instincts survived—I immediately started thinking about where I could find her a heavy winter coat, boots, hat, and gloves to protect her from the sub-zero temperatures.

Elizabeth mercifully spared me from questions about what I had done, why I had done it or how badly she felt because of my selfish actions. Her take-charge demeanor signaled to the nurses and to my twenty-four-hour suicide watch guard that their jobs might be a little easier thanks to her arrival.

Between my roommate's sisters and my little girl's optimistic, hopeful energy, our hospital room suddenly felt like a college dormitory on Move-In Day.

An unexpected visit from a hospital administrator the next day reinforced my relief at Elizabeth's presence. A pert young woman dressed in civilian clothes arrived with several papers—papers I mistook for release documents, since by that time I felt stable enough to go home.

It surprised me to hear her explain with the efficiency of a bank teller, "No, Mrs. Rhodes, these aren't for your discharge. We have to transfer you to another unit in the hospital for continued observation." She spread open the file folder with several pages neatly clipped together and flagged with yellow Post-it notes. "I'll need your signature here, here, and here so we can move you just as soon as a bed is ready for you on Reiss 2."

Had I actually grasped the gravity of what she was asking me to do and had I not been so intimidated by her enthusiastic, patronizing approach, I would have insisted that a lawyer review the papers first. As she waved a pen in my face, a faint internal alarm prompted me to react with questions instead of my trusting signature.

"Why do I need to be moved at all? I'm perfectly comfortable in this room, and I actually feel much better, and maybe I'm even okay to be released when my husband gets here later, so he can just take me home."

Her tightening lips revealed mounting impatience.

"You came in through the emergency room, Mrs. Rhodes. The hospital has to make sure you are well enough to leave and they won't know that until the doctors observe you for a few more days."

It seemed reasonable and I had no objection to staying as long as I needed care. But an uneasy feeling began gnawing at my gut as her arms crossed her expanding chest with exasperation. Suddenly this nice girl didn't seem so nice to me. I looked deeper into her eyes, trying to read her face for a hint of what was really going on.

"Maybe I should have my husband look at these papers anyway when he comes in later today. We'll go over them and decide what to do then."

"Mrs. Rhodes, I'm sorry but you don't really have a decision to make. If you refuse to sign these papers, the hospital has the legal right to automatically confine you at their own discretion in light of the circumstances. Remember, you did come in through the emergency room and you did try to take your life."

Suddenly my naiveté and imagined options morphed into a chilling awakening. Oh my God—I'm theirs until further notice. I'm not going anywhere they don't decide for me. What have I gotten myself into?

Elizabeth shared my consternation when she echoed my questions to the young woman hoping to gain further clarification, but with no success. We both looked helplessly at each other as I signed the papers with my right hand, fingers crossed on my left.

She left the room as Elizabeth and I brushed off our mistrustful hunches, obediently settling into a few days' wait for transfer to my new room on what the staff referred to as a non-medical floor. Why I didn't twitch at the reference to "non-medical floor" confounds me now. I suppose it's because I had absolutely no idea that it was code for "psych ward." Nor did I have even the slightest suspicion of what lay in store for me once they wheeled me through the maze of hospital corridors and left me behind the securely locked doors of Reiss 2.

3 | Welcome to the Psych Ward

Alice: *But I don't want to go among mad people.*
The Cat: *Oh, you can't help that. We're all mad here.*
I'm mad. You're mad.
Alice: *How do you know I'm mad?*
The Cat: *You must be. Or you wouldn't have come here.*

— Lewis Carroll, *Alice in Wonderland*

If Elizabeth hadn't flown up from Florida and stayed by my side, I'd expect my description of what happened with my transfer to the psychiatric ward—known as Reiss 2—would be chalked up to a crazy woman's exaggerated perceptions.

Five days after my arrival at Saint Vincent's, by 6:00 pm on Monday evening, Elizabeth tucked me and my few personal belongings into a wheelchair. She held my hand as the orderly set us in motion down the brightly lit corridor into a cavernous elevator. I had no idea where we were going—other than the people in charge of my recovery unanimously decided I needed "to be moved."

We silently meandered through the maze of halls connecting the hospital's obvious stages of development from modern new wings to an older, almost antique-like ambiance. It felt good to have a change of scenery from the previous week's confinement in the Coleman medical wing's routines. As we passed through the original hospital's entrance lobby, the old-fashioned incandescent fixtures cast a dimmed reverence on the frozen-faced founders' portraits along the mahogany-paneled walls. Vintage guest chairs, elegantly upholstered in worn leather and tapestry, now sat as evidence to a smaller, more intimate and welcoming hospital, long ago displaced by the modern institution's hustle and bustle. I detected the scent of burning church candles even before we passed the heavy oak doorway to the chapel. As we wheeled past the plaster statues of Catholic saints flanking the entrance, I winced at my lapsed Catholic status and wondered if my suicide attempt had sealed my destiny to Hell's eternal flames.

Our excursion ended as a heavy metal door loudly slammed behind us with an unfamiliar but disturbingly recognizable finality. The attendant delivered me in my wheelchair to a floor with the exact opposite feeling of the Coleman medical unit's brightly lit, comforting patient care atmosphere. With a tacit nod he released my papers to a severe-faced nurse as I peered over the top of the bag of personal belongings filling my lap. Although trying to assess the nature of my new surroundings, the realization that this was a bona fide psychiatric ward still hadn't dawned on me. Not until the first series of blood curdling screams filled the hall did I begin to comprehend I was in a situation I'd only read about in novels or seen in scary movies.

A stench of urine, murky halls with ominous inmates' silhouettes hovering and then shuffling along in hospital garb with their naked backsides exposed, and the muffled sounds of groans echoing in the background immediately informed us we were in the wrong place. Someone in the front office must have made a mistake. The orderly got the papers mixed up and delivered me to the wrong floor.

As the ear-bending screams continued, Elizabeth and I took seats in beat-up plastic chairs directly across from the doorway we had just crossed. Our eyes locked in stunned silence. Before we had a chance to murmur our concerns to each other, a thickset woman dressed in a hospital uniform concealed by an oversized, mossy green sweater approached. A note of caution subtly laced her voice as she directed me to a room further down the corridor from where we were sitting.

"I don't think we should go any further with my transfer because I won't be staying. I'd like to find another floor either in this hospital or in another—but this place is too scary for me to handle."

My bold naiveté either confirmed how crazy I was or gave this woman material for a shared laugh at the nurses' station. Without missing a beat, without even a blink of acknowledgment to my protests, she shook her head. "Mrs. Rhodes, you will be staying here tonight and until I receive a release from your doctor," (whoever that was—I had been seen by several) "we will proceed with your intake process."

Dumbfounded and impotent, I got up from the chair and followed her alone down the dimly lit hall into a room with an overhead light that exposed the cold, stark reality of my circumstances. I looked around the room, bewildered and without an ounce of strength to question anything. I needed a few moments to assess what was actually happening to me. It felt as if I had taken a wrong turn and my internal GPS automatically complained, "Recalculating!"

She instructed me to strip naked.

"Even my underwear?" I asked as I stood shivering in the middle of the room.

"Yes, I have to see everything."

She sat in a chair making notes on a form as she examined every inch of my skin for identifying scars, marks of self-injury, rash, disease, evidence of hypodermic drug use and whatever other dermatological secrets psych patients might conceal. She made sure my hair and scalp were lice-free and my mouth was checked for God-knows-what. Another barrage of questions came flying.

"Are you hearing voices? Do you fear someone is trying to harm you? Are you seeing things that aren't there?"

I answered "No" to everything, all the while worried that this nurse believed I was a bona fide psycho and my responses didn't matter, regardless of their veracity.

I dressed my now-surrendered body as she handed me a two-page copy of the house rules and regulations while informing me that my cell phone and all personal belongings would be confiscated and secured at the nurses' station until my departure. This included any and all items with stiff, sharp protruding edges, as well as anything else that could be used as a weapon. She apologized that I had missed the dinner hour but assured me that my room, with a strange but harmless roommate, would be ready for me as soon as my paperwork was complete. I walked out of the examination in a quiet but festering rage—frustrated, helpless, frightened, and utterly confounded.

Elizabeth dutifully remained where I had left her by the locked door, tears streaming down her beautiful face. "Mom, I can't leave you here. You can't stay here. We have to get you out of here!"

I agreed but spoke with a surprisingly calm stoicism, prompting her to ask me, "Mom, are you scared? Because you don't look like you're scared, but this place is really awful."

I replied with a mask-like demeanor. "Honey, what you are looking at is my game face."

We sat in stunned silence for the next half hour, taking in the demented ambiance of the Reiss 2 Welcoming Committee.

When a young aide finally escorted me to my room, Elizabeth left me with the promise that she would find a way to get me out. My lingering gratitude for the hope she imparted for the both of us became my only connection with reality. In the meantime I had to get through the night alone, cold, unfed, and unsure of how I would ever come out the other end of this unfathomable situation.

My room was every bit as austere as the intake room. Overhead lighting, linoleum floor, two very small, wooden beds (mine with no blanket) and a flat, lifeless pillow. Bare walls, not a mirror in sight. Great care was taken to ensure that no cord, screw, or piece of glass or plastic could be misappropriated for self-harm. The large single window looked out into a four-sided, brick-lined cavern. The adjoining bathroom contained a mold-infested shower with no shower curtain and disgusting clumps of dark hair covering the floor and drain. The toilet was replete with errant pubic hairs, dried urine, and crusted feces. Soap, shampoo, towels and such were nowhere in sight. I found out later that if I needed any supplies they were available down the hall in a locked laundry room. It must have been assumed I should have the common sense to ask, but then common sense was the least of my abilities at this point.

My security blanket became a small, handmade quilt I had won in an auction at a non-profit fund-raiser a few months earlier. John had brought it to me during my earlier stay on the medical floor. Having something that was made with careful, loving hands to use as a pillow and personal coverlet assuaged my fretful heart.

As it was February and one of the coldest winter weeks on record, news reports bemoaned how even the mightiest furnaces struggled to provide adequate comfort throughout the city. This wing of the hospital was no exception. The ceilings in my room were at least twelve feet high, making the four walls surrounding me feel even colder. Staring blankly and trying to comprehend the scope of my predicament, I sat on the edge of my bed facing the drafty window, afraid to move even a pinky finger.

One of the house rules required that all doors must remain open. No click of a door handle, not even a squeak of a hinge warned me when my roommate crept in—a small, older woman with unruly white hair. Her unexpected appearance unnerved me almost as much as her inability to speak or understand a word of English—which I discovered when she began ranting at me for what reason I will never know. I found out later she was a permanent resident at Reiss 2, a "regular," one of the club members. Being a rookie myself, I didn't feel I had the prerogative to leave the light on when she wanted to go to sleep, albeit at 8:00 pm. In a state of incredulity I sat ramrod straight in complete darkness on the edge of my bed, continuing to stare out the viewless window. I tried desperately to tune out my roommate's cacophonous snoring just a few feet away, but I was riveted in place by the incessant screaming coming from somewhere down the hall.

Periodically, a patrol person would stop by to peer in and make sure we were still there. I kept my back to the door, ignoring them, but their padded footsteps told me they had me in their sights. Passersby drifted along in the hallway throughout the night as I watched their reflections appear in my TV-screen of a window. The longer I sat there the more frozen I became, not from the bitter cold air coming in through the drafty window but by the feeling of sheer terror slipping itself around my neck like a noose on a gallows. I couldn't breathe, I couldn't think, I couldn't sleep. The insane screaming of some tortured soul persisted throughout the night with the accompanying fulminations of a man spewing obscenities well into the early morning hours. Fear continued to envelop me as I wildly fantasized someone slipping into the room to either physically attack me or, at the very least, choose me as a new victim to bellow at. After all, I was in the midst of crazy people, wasn't I?

It soon became a game of wills for me. Over and over I silently repeated to myself: I will stay awake no matter what. I will not give in to sleep. I will show them how I can stick it out no matter what and sleep isn't going to slip me up and allow me to succumb to any of this madness.

I won the game. It would be another fifty-two hours before I would be able to finally close my eyes and sleep.

A lighter view of the alleyway emerged as the night hours transformed into morning. An attendant came around looking for my blood pressure reading and blood and urine samples, which I refused to give. Since my plan was still in place to leave, I saw no need to participate in any other procedure. She duly noted this in her book and subsequently reported it to the head nurse.

I was busted for resisting the morning routine but the head nurse's admonitions to cooperate only reinforced my resolution about not spending another hour in this place. This also included refusing breakfast, as that meant I would have to sit in the dining area with the crazy people.

"Well, you'll have to explain all this to Dr. G and his staff at morning rounds later. They'll want to know why you won't eat and they'll definitely take action about needing your blood and urine samples."

"I'm not worried about explaining anything. My family is coming to take me home today, anyway." I did my best to remain as unemotional as possible but underneath I started to feel the nagging doubt that real fear can incite. We concluded an amicable standoff—for the time being.

Earlier that morning Elizabeth had left a message with the nurses that she and John were securing a bed for me at a private hospital in Connecticut much closer to home. They had set the wheels in motion to get pre-approval from the insurance company. I remained as optimistic as humanly possible, relying on this bit of second-hand encouragement as a substitute for the energy a good night's sleep and a hot breakfast would have otherwise provided.

Besides, I needed to prepare my case for my meeting with the attending physicians that morning. I needed to be ready to explain my situation: that I didn't belong here and that I wanted the proper documents signed by the doctors so I could leave.

∾∾

"Rounds" on Reiss 2 was a forum where the head of the psychiatric unit sits with resident doctors who are learning the tricks of the psychiatric trade. When my turn came, the nurse's aide fetched me from my room and guided me across the hall to a small meeting room jammed full with chairs lining three walls. About sixteen students sat elbow-to-elbow, laps piled high with heavy, manila file folders. Their collective stare was palpable. I took the obvious single chair on the fourth wall, tacitly reserved for the patient of the hour. I couldn't tell if they were curious, thirsty-for-knowledge students or garden variety shrinklettes-in-training.

There was no mistaking the alpha dog in this pack, however. Dr. G exuded the aura of a presiding Lord-High-Everything with a gratuitous, inflated, and officious demeanor. I felt hung like the target at a local turkey shoot as his sycophants competed with one another, taking turns aiming textbook questions at me—did I understand what I did, what did I think about what I did, would I try to do it again—on and on, caring more about impressing their leader than any answer I could offer.

My game face firmly in place, I took a deep breath and explained with great remorse how I understood what I'd done was wrong, and how the preceding night on the ward had been very frightening and I needed to be in a place where I felt safer. I emphatically explained that my devoted and resourceful family had contacted a private hospital in Connecticut with an available bed, and we were now just waiting for the okay from Saint Vincent's so I could transfer. These princes of mental health care met my plan with a mixture of seat-squirming, leg-crossing, eye-averting, and heads-bowed-down note taking, and nary a soul in the room indicated even a glimmer of understanding, empathy, or assent.

I took my cue to leave the room when Dr. G curtly nodded and slapped my file folder shut. As I reached the door, he made it crystal clear to me that my release depended on his and his colleagues' opinions about my condition. My personal preference as to where I recuperated had no influence on the matter whatsoever. A sinking feeling that things were not going as I hoped followed me out the door. I had no experience in the mental health care world and I knew I needed some serious help.

Desperation set in as I waited my turn to use the public telephone on the wall in the corridor outside my room. The moment had arrived for me to go into a dial-a-thon to find someone who could help me get out of Reiss 2, someone who would understand that although I knew I needed dedicated psychiatric care, I couldn't possibly heal in a place that was so unhealthy, both physically and emotionally.

I called John, who had spent the morning with Elizabeth on the phone making arrangements for my transfer. He confirmed that we were all set to go to the hospital in Connecticut—close to home and covered by our insurance. Increasingly worried about Dr. G's parting caution as I left the morning rounds, I called my sister who worked in the health care non-profit world for advice about my legal rights; I called another friend who had just finished an advanced nursing program, looking for ways to position my plea in case Dr. G could actually stop my transfer; I scoured my brain trying to think of anyone who could possibly influence the guards of Saint Vincent's who held the keys to my fate. The bed at the Connecticut hospital had my name on it for only twenty-four hours. The pressure was on for me to make this transfer happen.

My next opportunity to meet with the doctors at rounds wouldn't happen for another twenty-four hours. I remained wide awake with no hope for even a wink of sleep and no appetite for food, the smell of which only intensified the nausea overtaking my stomach. I decided compliance with the rules was a better course for release, so I stood on line that afternoon and evening for vitals readings.

My blood pressure, registered at 97/64 when I left the medical unit, now clocked in at 160/98. As long as my blood pressure remained so drastically above normal, the doctors considered me to be at risk. I presumed this was another deterring factor in gaining my release. I couldn't win for losing, The stress of the environment caused my abnormally high blood pressure, prolonging my confinement, but if I could only get out of there, I knew it would return to its usual, healthy, "lower than normal" status.

My mind's strategy wheels churned as an escape plan took shape.

∾

The population mix on Reiss 2 consisted of a combination of young substance abusers caught in compromising situations in the outside world and who ended up in the hospital, joined by a community of geriatric patients suffering from dementia and other mental disorders that accompany old age. Most of the latter signed on as indigent cases whose medical bills were covered by the state or federal government. Few to almost none of them had any family on hand. The surrealism of the place lent itself to my own cinematic fantasy. Central Casting's job would have been a slam-dunk if they showed up on the ward looking for extras.

We were expected to dine and spend time in the community room, away from the isolation of our rooms. I had no interest in socializing since—with the tunnel vision of a pro golfer on the eighteenth hole—I focused on being able to transfer out. I allowed no distractions from my mission to find a way out of Reiss 2. In the meantime, Elizabeth dependably showed up that morning with the *New York Times* and accompanying cups of darkly brewed coffee that we shared in the farthest corner of the common room. I took my meal trays to this now-established personal post and discovered that the patients and staff in the common room seemed willing to grant me my space without censure. It became my private office where I visited with my family and, most important, my assigned and dedicated social worker, Josh.

Josh's office was on the same floor as the ward, but he would seek out and meet with his cases wherever he could locate them during the day. He could always find me at my corner table, and Elizabeth and I made sure he knew how desperately I needed his help. After my initial meeting with Josh when I explained my desire to move to another hospital closer to home—and clearly one that had a reputation for being quite the antithesis of Reiss 2—he pled my case to the director of Saint Vincent's psychiatric department, the very same honcho doctor whose approval I failed to gain at the previous day's rounds meeting. Unfortunately, Josh faced the same wall of resistance from Dr. G with no explanation. I was under the big boss's care until further notice.

After my second morning's failed tribunal and Josh's unsuccessful lobbying efforts on my behalf, Elizabeth, John, and I insisted on meeting with the good doctor to try to understand what level of "okay-ness" I needed to achieve in order for him to sign a transfer form.

"What is it you need to see before you'll allow Martha to transfer?" John asked in his usual measured and reasonable tone. Elizabeth sat with all her senses fired up and ready for battle. I might as well have been in a courtroom sitting between my two defense lawyers, silent and fearful of the verdict.

Dr. G's reply sounded vague and obtuse. "The other resident doctors just aren't comfortable with releasing you to another hospital" was the only answer he could offer.

The only discomfort I discerned was in his body language, which showed marked uneasiness when we pressed him with very logical, legitimate questions regarding his and the others' concerns. The underarms of his dress shirt became increasingly wet with perspiration. His hands gestured in mid-air as if he were an untrained orchestra conductor. He even posed the scenario that I might flee from the ambulance while being transported to another hospital. We quickly offered that I could be strapped down to prevent any malfeasance on my part, but evidently he perceived me to be a woman with Houdini in my DNA who would contrive a way to escape.

As our meeting came to a close I knew my day in this psych ward would end with me still in captivity. His parting words of self-justification to us were simply, "Look, you should be happy, this is the nice floor!" I subsequently discovered there were two other psychiatric units at Saint Vincent's harboring severely impaired psychotic patients and deranged social reprobates. As far as I was concerned, my fate lay in the least of three evils, but there was absolutely nothing nice about Reiss 2 for me at that moment.

It didn't take me long to figure out how to play the game in this new world of mine. I managed to get my room assignment changed to one with a window that faced West Twelfth Street. As I peered out through the heavy-gauged grate covering the window, I observed people bundled up in winter coats as they hustled along to the business of their lives. My new reality stung me like a bitter, cold wind. *That used to be me.* I started to panic. I felt like a prisoner with no voice, wanting to scream out to them, "Please, come and save me! I'm being held against my will and there's no way out!" Of course they wouldn't hear me and, even if they did, I was in a psych ward so my pleas would be for naught. Incredibly, my mind wondered how I, Martha Rhodes, a woman of resources both intellectual and physical, could be embroiled in what had become, in my mind, a serious hostage situation. How did I ever get here? Why didn't I know what it meant to be in a mental hospital? Hadn't I seen enough movies and plays about this? *One Flew Over the Cuckoo's Nest* or *Girl, Interrupted*?

Suddenly, the fiction I knew in the past became frighteningly real to me now. I expected my hospitalization to start the healing process for a very serious illness. Instead, my hospital stay seemed to be nothing more than a holding pen for patients who don't know how to live life normally. There was no healing going on. There was no therapy, no treatment, no counseling with a doctor to help me understand what had happened to me and how I could possibly move forward with my life. It was a place for stabilizing the unstable, at which point the newly aligned psychos would be released either to their own devices or, if lucky, to some form of outpatient group care.

When the assigned student psychiatrist appeared in my room to let me know that consideration for my release wouldn't happen for at least another four days, my game face evaporated and I completely fell apart, a collapsed pile of tears on the bed. I begged her to understand how scared and unhappy I felt in Reiss 2 and how much better the hospital in Connecticut would be, not only for me but for my family whom I desperately needed to have near me now and who had to drive so far into New York to be with me.

I regained my composure when I realized she was dead serious and looking her straight in the eye I said, "I just want you to know this place is a hell hole." With a response as frozen as the icy street outside my window, her face was devoid of any compassion or understanding whatsoever. It struck me as odd that such a bright young woman who had chosen a field involving patient care could possibly remain so unmoved by another woman's desperate tears. I had done everything I knew to be compliant with the system: I spent the required hours outside of my room sitting quietly or interacting with others in the common room; I ate my meals in the dining room; I attended the group meetings intended for those with addictions; I willingly lined up for the daily vital signs check-in, and I even engaged other patients in conversation while watching TV in one of the lounges. My behavior was duly noted in the book in which the staff placed check marks in the appropriate columns on an hourly basis as to each patient's whereabouts. Too much time alone in your room was a "no-no." Not eating meals or refusing to offer up your arm for a blood pressure check got you a negative mark in the book.

It didn't take me but thirty-six hours to see that good behavior here was even more critical than when I sat at my desk in Sister Emily's fifth-grade class at Saint Augustine Catholic School. There, misbehavior had meant banishment to the cloakroom. Stepping out of line on Reiss 2 meant something far more ominous and frighteningly unknown. Suddenly those memories of the cloakroom seemed like a vacation in comparison. At least there I knew a bell would ring and my class, including me, would be dismissed.

Around the third day of confinement, Josh offered me the locations and phone numbers for the New York State Office of Mental Health, the New York State Department of Health, the New York State Joint Commission, and the New York State Hospital Code Section 405.7 which explained in detail the Patient's Bill of Rights pertaining to confinement in a mental institution.

Furthermore, he provided me with contact information for an attorney who was available to patients in need of legal counsel and representation in cases such as mine. I quickly reviewed the Patient's Rights document and got on the phone with him to explain the situation as I understood it at the time. He listened attentively and agreed to investigate and call me later. On the surface he could see no reason I should not be allowed to transfer to another hospital. He knew it and I knew it. So did the social worker. So did some of the nurses on the floor.

I discovered sometime later that the only problem in transferring me was the issue of the quota of bodies in beds at Saint Vincent's Hospital, keeping their financial bottom line alive—and my pitiful butt was part of that number. As long as they could bill my insurance company for my hospital stay, taking my business elsewhere was out of the question.

As caring and concerned as the staff tried to be, my intuition picked up an undercurrent of discontent within the staff's ranks as the days wore on. Some staff members were totally sterile, "by the book" caretakers. And there were others who were well-trained, compassionate caregivers. Their demeanor toward me and some of the other patients made it obvious to which camp each belonged.

I also knew that none of them had an easy job and, by the time I thought I would hate them all, I managed to find a place in my heart to admire them, to be grateful to them for the difficult job they faced each day, and to respect the seemingly idiotic rules they enforced for the sake of the greater good on the floor. I wasn't looking to make their job any harder—I just wanted to get the hell out of their workplace. I believe some of them came to realize my genuine appreciation for what they had to do, as well as how unnecessary it was for me to be grouped in with the caliber of insane patients currently on the floor. I'm sure the scuttlebutt among them included my persistent appeals to Dr. G for my transfer, as well as my pursuit of legal channels to dispute his intractable position.

Already armed with the Patients' Bill of Rights and legal aid information, I found out that as a voluntary patient I had the right to submit a written request to leave the hospital. Upon doing so, I must be released within seventy-two hours unless the Director of the Psychiatry believed I met the requirements for involuntary admission and therefore needed to stay. Under this law the director has the same seventy-two hours to apply for authorization to a judge to keep the patient. I quickly wrote a request on a sheet torn from a small notebook and handed it to the head nurse. As a savvy businesswoman in the past, I at least had the wherewithal to know that without a copy to prove its existence, my request stood the chance of dropping down a bottomless black hole.

"May I please have a copy of my letter?" I asked.

The charge nurse curtly responded, "The hospital doesn't make copies."

My distrust and disbelief became evident to everyone in the nurses' station, including a clerical aide who quietly took my original. Under her breath she gently assured me, "I'll make you one a little later when we're not so busy." Wide-eyed, I gratefully backed off my insistent position.

On the sly, this benevolent woman pulled a photocopy, folded it up in her uniform pocket and surreptitiously slipped it to me a few hours later as I sat at my table in the common room. To avoid exposing her, I nervously stuck it under my shirt, as if we were executing a high-profile espionage tactic. By now I began to suspect that if I wasn't completely crazy when I arrived on this floor, certifiable insanity lurked just around the corner.

These sorts of antics chipped away at any sense of reality I so desperately needed to hold onto. But with the covert support I received from the nurse's aide, I began to feel as if I were being secretly cheered on as the leading role in the movie, *David Meets Goliath On Reiss 2*. Here was a patient willing to challenge the great Dr. G, king of the psychiatric hill. Here was a patient who knew her rights (barely) and was exercising them.

My emotional and mental state prevented me from seeing any positive actions on my part at the time and, truth to tell, I felt like a pitiful, vulnerable waif in the scheme of things, unable to fend for myself as I normally would. In retrospect, I know now that I had successfully "made friends and influenced people" when an angel of a nurse came to my room to let me know it was lunchtime. She discovered me weeping after my last hope of leaving anytime soon was crushed by the resident doctor, who had just told me I would be staying until the following week.

As I tried to explain to her why I was so distraught, she comforted me with her kindly Irish brogue and in frustration blurted out, "I don't know why he has you staying here either! None of us do. You don't belong here if you've got a hospital closer to home!"

I lifted my head from my lap and leapt into her arms. Finally, I had someone who got it that I was in the wrong place. I hugged her and thanked her for seeing what I really needed. I started crying all over again, not with tears of hopelessness and desperation, but with tears of gratefulness and relief.

The rest of that day and evening, I pulled myself together for no other reason than I knew someone had my back. I wasn't alone and I would make it through no matter what. I finally catnapped for a few hours. I enjoyed a couple of TV shows with other patients as we talked about the characters and tried to second-guess the plot. That night the staff served ice cream in the common room—I had two helpings. The check marks under my name in the book were lining up nicely. I proved to everyone and to myself what a good citizen I could be. Two other patients had fulfilled their five-day incarceration sentence and left earlier that afternoon. I knew them only briefly, but nevertheless, seeing them go moved me for some strange reason. Maybe I felt a hint of jealousy, a feeling of being left behind, or perhaps just a basic sadness that they had to be there in the first place.

As I took my seat at the breakfast table the next morning, the same nurse with the Irish accent tapped me on the shoulder from behind and whispered in my ear, "Don't worry anymore, Dearie, you're going to be leaving here sometime today." My breath escaped me and it didn't come back until I digested what she had actually said to me. I wondered if I had heard her correctly. She didn't go into any details as she whisked herself out of the room. She obviously had a clandestine mission, and further conversation with me could have derailed her efforts.

Later in the day I received a report that this courageous nurse had gone above the head of Dr. G and informed the director of nursing about my case. The next thing I knew, my social worker visited me, all aflutter with faxes and papers to sign, lining up the proper documents for the Connecticut hospital and arranging for transportation to get me there. It would be just a matter of time to arrange all the pieces for my exodus.

The afternoon crawled by, even though the student nurses completing their psychiatric care training module threw a little party for the inmates with music, chips, and soda for the occasion. The festivities provided me with a much-needed distraction as my excitement about leaving mounted with each passing minute.

I abandoned my secluded, back corner table and took a seat on one of the upholstered couches among the other patients. A faint odor of old urine mixed with disinfectant enveloped me, but I was able to inhale and exhale with ease knowing it would be my last day in the community room.

I noticed one old man whom I'd never heard speak a word or had even seen him smile, and who never had any visitors. His dark skin rested in little ripples on his bony arms protruding from a well-worn tee shirt. He had large, vacant eyes set inside deep sockets and a high forehead. He seemed content enough sharing a spot at a long table with a nursing student, a paper plate filled with orange cheese snacks within easy reach, staring into space and leaving me to wonder if he even knew what was going on around him. I felt pity for him, imagining his destiny sealed in this lonely world of disability and dysfunction.

In an effort to properly entertain the man, the student experimented with different CDs, playing a sampling of rock 'n' roll, country, and popular light music.

"Do you like this one, Carl?" No comment from Carl.

"How about this one?" Still no reaction.

She appeared to be close to giving up when she inserted a third CD into the portable boom box and hit the play button. Suddenly an enormous, white-toothed smile broke through Carl's blank expression. His lifeless arms lifted from his lap. His eyes opened and lit up as his shiny head bobbed back and forth to the music—and he began scat singing to Sam Cooke's "You Send Me" with the improvisational familiarity of a seasoned jazz musician. When the song finished, Carl resumed his original vacuous state. I couldn't take my eyes off him as I sat in wonderment, marveling at music's universal ability to transform even the weariest of souls, including my own.

A bell rang signaling all the residents elsewhere on the ward to gather in the common room. The head nurse stood in the center of the floor and waited for everyone's attention.

"I'd just like to thank our graduating students for their fine work over the past eight weeks, and for hosting this lovely party for our patients."

The students stood in a line side-by-side and wrapped their arms around each other's waist, their faces flushed with exhaustion or pride—I couldn't tell which. Everyone applauded and nodded their heads in appreciation, but I got the impression these festivities occurred every few weeks with the same formula of chips, soda, and boom box music as another crop of students came and went.

The head nurse continued. "We are delighted you are moving on in your medical careers and wish you all the best. And speaking of moving on, one of our patients will be leaving us today—Martha."

I never expected my departure to be made public—as if I had done something wonderful to deserve the honor of recognition. My plan was to sneak out under a veil of secrecy and never look back. Her announcement stunned me. I sat there mute and self-conscious until I spotted two women who seemed to have taken a liking to me during our brief time together during meals, meetings and TV time. Their faces drooped with disappointment at the news. I felt sorry for them because I knew they wouldn't get out of there any time soon. They were pretty hard cases. Nothing I could say or do would change their circumstances, nor did I want to show my elation about leaving Reiss 2 for fear of rubbing salt into the wound of their abandoned feelings. I quietly thanked everyone and left it at that.

High spirits continued to waft for the remainder of the afternoon as I patiently awaited my release. The already gray day grew darker as the dinner hour approached. Brief goodbye visits from my newfound friends on the ward bolstered my belief that I would be leaving before the day was done, but with every passing hour my confidence in my captors' ability to sort out the red tape began to wane. I scoured my memory trying to recall the last time, if ever, anyone held my fate so tightly in his grip.

By six o'clock that evening my escape car finally arrived. As the uniformed EMTs strapped me onto the stretcher and moved me out into the fresh air of the West Village into the ambulance, I urged myself to "just be in the moment"—something I had never ever truly done until that exact, free and clear instant.

Almost seventy-two hours to the minute had transpired since I entered the world of Reiss 2. It felt like seventy-two years.

～

For all the times I had driven into New York City as a commuter, speeding past the view on the West Side Highway, it seemed sadly ironic to be sitting in the rear of an ambulance experiencing the same view facing backward and moving in reverse. I'd never been in an emergency vehicle in my life. The smell of the cabin and the sounds of the equipment bumping around as the van made its way through the heavy rush hour traffic distracted me while I settled in for the long ride.

The driver's co-pilot, a hefty young woman, gave me the impression she needed to get in tight with her partner. Although she took her place in the back next to me, she completely ignored me as she leaned over the front seat, feeding him the latest tidbits of cool pop culture. I doubted if even a sudden bout of vomiting or spontaneous bleeding would have grabbed her attention.

A sense of invisibility shifted to vulnerability as I now had an hour and a half to imagine what might be in store for me at Silver Hill Hospital in Connecticut. My intense mission to get out of Saint Vincent's had obscured any feelings of either excitement or anxiety from surfacing—until now. It occurred to me that I might be jumping from the frying pan into the fire.

How did I even get here in this ambulance on my way to another loony bin? And when I get there in an hour, will I start feeling better or will I go further down the rat hole? Will anyone at Silver Hill actually care if I live or die, or will I be given another bed to while away the time until I seem fit for living again? Will I be locked up like a criminal to protect me from myself or will I be given a warm and sympathetic therapist who will ask me the sixty-four thousand dollar question, "Why did you do this to yourself, Martha?" *and will anyone be able to help me figure out the answer?*

I felt like a stranger to myself, bouncing around hospitals among other strangers. I didn't understand what was expected of me and how the psychiatric care system was supposed to work. I was on a steep learning curve in "Suicide 101."

The ambulance deftly weaved in and out of the traffic as we

melded with the mass of commuters heading for home. Headlights from the cars behind us intermittently flashed across my face through the van's rear windows as I sentimentally fantasized about the commuters' push to get home to their loved ones after a hard day's work in the big city. I used to be one of them, anxious to shed the city's stress and fall into my suburban home's familiar comfort. I idealistically assumed everyone anticipated where they were going and who would welcome them when they got there.

Everyone—except for me.

4 | OUT OF THE OCEAN, ONTO THE SHORE

"No matter where you go—there you are."

– Confucius

New Canaan, Connecticut is a quaint New England bedroom community primarily suited for New York financial moguls. It's the town next to where my husband teaches school and has always held a certain mystique for me, given its affluence and country club atmosphere. A regular car route to and from activities in that neck of the woods frequently put me at an intersection where I always noticed a small, wrought iron sign discreetly lettered with the words "Silver Hill." Not Silver Hill Hospital, not Silver Hill Psychiatric Clinic and Rehabilitation Center. Just a sweet, classy, metal sign and an equally understated arrow pointing in the direction of the grounds that lay somewhere up the long, country road, back behind the trees. Almost as if to say, "You have to come look for Silver Hill, it doesn't go looking for you."

I spotted this plaque nestled among the roadside trees countless times over the past thirty-five years, unable to resist a morbid fascination about Silver Hill's secrets. I'd heard that only rich people went there, celebrities who could easily afford the rent and could ill afford the publicity. It carried an aura of supreme privacy and elitism. It was "the" place to land if you had a problem with alcoholism, drug addiction, nervous breakdown, or any other troubles of the rich and famous.

John made the arrangements for me to transfer from Reiss 2 at Saint Vincent's to Silver Hill. I wondered how painful it must have been for him to make those calls. Now, instead of coming home on the commuter railroad, I arrived in an ambulance. For over twenty years John had waited for me to return to Connecticut after a long day's work in the city. He'd listened for the train's whistle as it pulled into the station close to our home and zipped down the road to pick me up. He'd always welcomed me with the warmest embrace— unfailingly upbeat and genuinely happy to have me home. My arrival this night bore no resemblance to those other receptions.

As the attendants angled the transport stretcher into the reception building, I spotted John sitting alone in the waiting area, staring blankly at the carpeted floor. A brief phone call from the social worker in New York alerted him that I would be leaving Saint Vincent's around six o'clock, but rush hour traffic delayed my arrival in Connecticut until 8:00 pm. He'd been there for over an hour with plenty of time to worry and plan for the next phase of the nightmare consuming our lives. The commotion from the stretcher wrested him from his stupor. He got up and came into the hall where the ambulance attendant deposited me and my belongings. The other attendant reported to someone in an adjoining room with the same familiarity a UPS deliveryman greets customers on his daily route. Their mission accomplished, they wished me luck and left. I was signed for and delivered.

I gingerly reached for John's arm as he guided me into a small, comfortable room with a lush carpet and antique, upholstered chairs where we were asked to wait.

"Hi, sweetheart, how was the ride and how're you feeling?"

I nodded and hugged him as if I'd just returned from a long trip to the other side of the world.

"Sit here next to me. There's tea, water, and snacks in the basket. Can I get you anything?"

"No, thanks. Let's just wait. I'm exhausted and I'm sure you are, too." I replied.

John's words reassured me that he still loved me but I sensed an unfamiliar caution. It had been over a week since he received the call that I was in Saint Vincent's emergency room. And although

44

the five days on the medical floor passed quietly with his daily visits, my following three days in the psychiatric ward had taken its toll on him. His exhaustion, his worry, and his helplessness hung off his shoulders like a ragged old coat.

I felt overwhelmed with gratitude for the herculean effort he had put into securing me a bed at Silver Hill and for delivering me from the throes of Reiss 2. Still, I would never in a million years have imagined myself in a reception room waiting to be admitted to Silver Hill. John and I sat side by side, wordless, our hands clasped together, dangling in mid-air over the chairs' arms. The only thing passing between us now was an intense sense of relief that we were together and I was closer to home, safe with the one person I knew I could entrust with my life.

Shortly before I met John, a psychic predicted I would meet the man of my dreams. "Everyone should have a love like this," she proclaimed over and over, repeatedly interrupting herself during our session as she connected with the spirits around her. At the time it all seemed like a girlish lark to me. Thirty-three years later, as I sat in the elegant chair that kept me comfortable while waiting for the intake assistant to fetch me, I remembered the psychic's words. Everyone should have a love like I shared with this man. I felt so grateful for him, and equally as sorry he got stuck with me. How could I have put him through such an ordeal? Why would anyone want to abandon so precious a love too few people ever know? Guilt singed my heart. Everyone should have a love like this. No one should have a wife like me.

Nearly an hour after my arrival, an efficient-looking young woman finally came out to the waiting room to begin the lengthy intake process. She noticed the handmade blanket I'd relied upon for security at Reiss 2 sitting on top of my bag and promptly told me I wouldn't be allowed to keep any personal items in my room.

"No special pillows, blankets, or stuffed animals. No pictures or little knickknacks." This policy seemed incongruous, since the place seemed so home-like and welcoming.

"May I keep my books?" I meekly asked.

"Yes, books are fine, but you'll be spending most of your time in group meetings so you won't need too many of them," she recited as we went into her inner office.

I sat next to her desk answering questions that by now seemed annoyingly routine to me—basic information such as name, address, age, insurance, and next of kin. She never once looked up at me as she tapped away on her computer keyboard faster than I could spit out the words. It hardly felt like a Kodak moment when she asked me to move in front of a blank wall where she snapped an identification photograph and attached it to my file.

Back in the reception area we waited until another aide escorted me to a room where I underwent an interview with a resident psychiatrist and submitted to a routine physical with another medical doctor. The questions reminded me of those asked at Saint Vincent's but, mercifully, they lacked the sharp edges. The psychiatrist told me he needed to determine whether I should be placed in an isolated, high-risk unit under lock and key with a 24/7 camera's eye on me, or if I could be trusted with my own safety and assigned a bed in the Main House where I would live in a more relaxed environment alongside other residents. The thought of being placed under lock and key again froze me. I had already convicted myself of an unforgivable offense. I knew they aimed to protect me from myself, but confining me to a solitary room would only serve to deepen my remorse. Having just escaped from a maximum-security situation and feeling anxious to prove my reliability to survive in a less restrictive setting, I answered their questions calmly and cautiously. My insightful approach got me a pass to the Main House. I felt relieved, but I took care not to appear overly excited for fear they might regard me as manic and renege on the offer. My game face remained in place until I could be sure of where I was going and what to expect.

I completed the intake process in one building and came

out to the reception room to kiss John good night. He looked exhausted. I couldn't tell if his eyes spoke more of sadness that he had to leave me again, or relief that I was finally closer to home and hopefully, closer to recovery.

"They're taking me to a room in the Main House. I'll be all right. Be careful driving home. It's late and you have to get up early for school tomorrow."

"Don't worry about me," he said. "Just get some rest."

We both felt awkward, but resigned to the next phase of this unfathomable situation. Confident I was now in caring and capable hands, John left for home with a promise to return the following day after school. I hoped his relief that he succeeded in getting me into a safe place would finally afford him a decent and well-deserved night's sleep.

∼∽

As I descended from the van that shuttled me across the grounds from the reception building to the Main House, I sucked in the cold, fresh, country air and held my face up toward the starlit sky. It revived me—invigorated me like a splash of cold, clear water. I confused its dark vastness with the ocean's, hardly able to distinguish between sea and sky, water and air. I felt like a tiny alien spec witnessing a world I no longer recognized. The young male attendant silently led the way as we climbed the wide stone steps to the tall front door of the Main House where I would spend my first night. As we entered the unlit entry hall, I peered to my left into what looked like a spacious living room. Expensive-looking draperies hung on the full-length windows. Classically upholstered love seats and wing back chairs were arranged in little clusters for intimate conversations. Although the lamps placed on polished mahogany tables throughout the room were dark, I noticed a tasteful shade atop each one.

"Wow, this place is gorgeous," I exclaimed.

"Yes they've just refurbished this building less than a year ago. You'll get a tour of the whole house tomorrow," the young man assured me.

Tomorrow. Never had the adage, "One day at a time" been more fitting. I couldn't think past the moment. The night was so dark and I was so exhausted that tomorrow seemed unreachable. In my gut I suddenly felt as if I had been plucked out of the middle of an angry ocean and plopped onto a very dry, safe shore.

We ascended a carpeted staircase to the second floor where the night shift nurse received me and immediately commandeered my bag of personal belongings. The lights in the eerily quiet and empty common area were dim. The adjoining nurses' station was even dimmer. At ten-thirty at night, I felt as if I were sneaking in after curfew.

"Hello, Martha. I'm Kathleen and I'll be taking you through the new patient orientation." Kathleen was a short, motherly woman who greeted me with a breathlessness befitting her full figure. She spoke with a hushed yet reassuring tone. My young escort quickly signed a slip she handed him and disappeared. She turned to me and recited our pending business at hand.

"First thing we have to do is go through your bag. We check for sharps and other banned materials and store them in a locker, but everything else will be returned to you in your room."

"And what's considered banned materials?" I asked.

"Oh, anything with alcohol in it—mouthwash, cologne, aftershave lotion. And, of course, any sharp objects like little scissors, nail clippers and files, compact powder cases with glass mirrors, and any glass cosmetic containers—here, like this one."

She discovered the thick, glass deodorant bottle in my cosmetics case.

"So this means I can't use deodorant while I'm here?"

"No, you just have to come to the storage area every morning and we'll hand it to you and then after you use it, put it back for safekeeping."

Ironically, I bought more expensive deodorant in a glass

bottle to save the environment from plastic. Now it was banned and confiscated to protect me from myself.

"Oh, and your cell phone. Patients aren't allowed to have cell phones—but don't worry, you'll get it back when you leave."

I'd forgotten I even had a cell phone. I hadn't spoken to anyone on it for over a week, nor did I care to at this point.

"Come with me, dear. We're going in here now." She led me to a little room with a small round table and two chairs just off the common area. "This won't take long. You've come to a wonderful place and I know everyone here will be looking after you. I'll leave you for a moment while you undress, and after your exam we'll get you settled in your room."

Almost three hours had transpired since my arrival from New York and I could see I wasn't even close to laying my head on a pillow. Although I had feared falling asleep at Saint Vincent's, I suddenly noticed the lack of it worked against me. I felt light-headed and punchy from the long ambulance ride and the lengthy intake examinations in the reception building. Now I still had to go through the mandatory body search and resident's orientation process.

This time, stripping down felt much less of an affront to my privacy. The carpeted floor provided warmth that made it feel more like a bedroom than an examination room. A minute or two later Kathleen politely tapped on the door. The fact that I could say, "Come in" made me feel as if I had a modicum of control, something I desperately missed during the past week.

She looked pleased to see that my hands didn't tremble when she asked me to extend my arms, and when I told her I didn't hear any strange voices she winked with a quick nod of her head. When she unwrapped the blood pressure cuff on my arm and announced my numbers—they were back to their normal low—I automatically returned the wink and the nod. This bit of information fortified my sense of safety and newly found security.

Kathy, as she by now wanted me to call her, showed me a small kitchenette and a coffeemaker ready for the next morning's brew.

"This is just for snacks. You'll be taking your main meals downstairs in the formal dining room. But just in case you're hungry in between or late at night, there's chips and cereal here in the cabinets, fruit, milk, and juice in the refrigerator.

"These two phones are for the patients. They come through the main phone system and only the people you wrote on your safe list will be put through. We write messages on this pad and post them here. If you hear the phone ring and you feel like picking it up, either call out for the person or take a message. They'll do the same for you." It all seemed so civilized and accommodating. This tiny bit of normal communication felt enormously encouraging.

Within the hour after my orientation, Kathy led me down a quiet hallway where she tucked me away in a warm corner room, the likes of which one might find in an upscale hotel—carpeted floor, soft ambient lighting, decorator-painted walls with a desk, chair, armoire, and a bed dressed with fluffy blankets, pillows, and my very own reading lamp built into the bed's headboard. Windows faced the spacious lawn I'd seen earlier from the shuttle van. Another door led to a clean, private bathroom, fitted with brand new fixtures, a tiled shower, plenty of thick towels, and a brightly lit mirror.

As I prepared myself for bed, I stood at the sink in front of the mirror. I hadn't seen my face since I left the medical floor at Saint Vincent's because Reiss 2 didn't allow mirrors. The person looking back at me took me by surprise. I hardly knew her. Her colorless complexion and limp hair showed no remnants of the smart, career-woman image I'd portrayed for over twenty years. The defeated, bewildered face stared at me, eyes aching with sadness. I wanted to look away, dismiss her like a bad dream, but I couldn't. Was it curiosity, self-pity, a sense of surrender, or perhaps a combination of those feelings that flooded my heart? As I look back, I think it was compassion that glued my gaze to the reflection. As I slowly brushed my teeth, the person in the mirror and I silently scrutinized each other, promising to become reacquainted.

~

My eyes opened slowly after my first peaceful night's sleep in over a week. The past twenty-four hours spent planning and executing my escape from Reiss 2 had been rife with anxiety, uncertainty, and desperation. The sound of chirping birds in the nearby trees that populated the picturesque grounds of Silver Hill made me wonder if I wasn't in a beautiful dream that had magically morphed from a nightmare of imprisonment and despair. The sense of relief filled every pore of my body and comforted me even more than the clean, fluffy blanket pulled up so snugly under my chin.

Before long, a staff person with the enthusiasm of a newly appointed camp counselor cracked open my closed door to inform me it was time to "rise and shine."

She let me know that missing breakfast was more than just breaking the rules, as she extolled the chef. "If you miss those yummy hotcakes you'll be madder than a wet hen!"

I quickly jumped into the spotless shower, the first time I had completely bathed myself in over a week since I left the Coleman medical floor at Saint Vincent's. The showers on Reiss 2 were a breeding ground for any number of contagious skin diseases, not to mention the fact that the water was never hot, not even warm, only tepid. I tried to be conservative with the length of my shower, but the act of cleansing myself took on a significance that nearly transfixed me standing there naked and wet.

"Wash away the past week of fear and frustration. Soap up and let those bubbles rejuvenate your spirit," I whispered aloud to myself. The thick, large white towel that embraced my exhausted body reassured me that today would indeed be a new day for a new life.

When John had met me at the registration building the night before, he brought a bag filled with clean, brightly colored blouses and fresh jeans, a much-needed change from the dreary black clothes that comprised my New-York-City, advertising-career wardrobe. A cozy, white cotton shawl speckled with primary colors eventually became my new security blanket. I wrapped myself up in it to cheer myself and soon discovered it provided cheer to others who saw me wearing it as well. John also brought me shampoo and other sorely missed toiletries to complete this extraordinary morning routine. A feeling of confidence carried me out the bedroom door and down the hall to the common area where the familiar aroma of freshly brewed coffee put a big smile on my face.

The morning schedule started upstairs with everyone's medications dispensed by a nurse through a little window, followed by vitals being recorded in another area of the common room. A few patients, who seemed to be already acquainted with one another, waited their turn for these procedures at a small, round table that lacked room for me to sit. They chatted over coffee and morning snacks available from the nearby kitchenette alcove.

A staff member introduced me as a new patient who had come in during the night. I felt uncomfortable and unsure if I should be too friendly in what was hardly a social gathering. I immediately recalled uncomfortable feelings of being an outsider in my high school lunchroom, where landing a seat at the table with the "in crowd" seemed like a lifetime goal. I wondered if I'd ever gotten over the anxiety of insecurity and feeling "less than." My life seemed like an unfulfilled quest for a sense of belonging. I never expected to belong in a psych hospital, however.

One of the younger women gently shifted her chair to the side and offered me a place with the group. I politely accepted the invitation.

"Good morning," I mumbled to a guy sitting across from me. The irony of the Stolichnaya logo on the left breast of his faded tee shirt didn't escape me. Yep, that's the vodka of choice, alright, I thought to myself. No one had a clue that I had swigged straight Stoli in order to down the bottle of Xanax tablets a week earlier. It felt good to see the humor in something for the first time in weeks—even black humor.

The common room I'd entered just a few hours earlier in darkness now appeared as a well-appointed, freshly painted, and comfortable facility. "Facility" almost seems an insult to describe it—it felt more like being in an elegant, expensive home.

Sunlight filled the room through an extra-long bay window running the entire length of the outside wall. The added bonus of a window seat below it invited patients to enjoy the view of the surrounding woods. Large upholstered chairs dotted the carpeted floor in front of a beautiful fireplace with a welcoming flagstone hearth. The nurses' station was discreetly incorporated into the floor plan where staff members performed their duties quietly and with a level of consummate respect for the patients.

Shortly after the morning meds and vitals were taken, everyone filed downstairs to the formal dining room. Other patients shared a variety of table arrangements, from settings for two or four to a long wooden table for a larger group to share their meal in lively conversation. I took a place at an empty table by myself in order to get a handle on the dining room dynamic. I needed to observe and assess how people interacted with each other before I could feel comfortable joining in. I wanted to be alone with my thoughts, alone with my confused feelings of relief and sadness.

Breakfast provided me with further comfort as the aromas from eggs, bacon, potatoes, fresh fruits and juices, yogurt, granola, pastries, and those acclaimed hotcakes grabbed my senses and wouldn't let go until the server on the buffet line had filled my plate twice with just about everything on the menu. I hadn't eaten in days and my appetite agreed with my heart that we were in an excellent place. The heat emanating through the china coffee mug warmed my hands as I digested not only the most delicious food

I had ever tasted in a setting where institutionally prepared food is notoriously poor, but also the realization that I was finally in a place where I could restart my mental and emotional engines. Everything I experienced at Silver Hill thus far had a recuperative, supportive feeling. I felt safe, clean, and hopeful.

The remainder of the first morning at Silver Hill required meeting with the entire medical/psychiatric staff in their daily ten o'clock rounds. I sat at the end of a long table answering questions similar to the ones asked at Saint Vincent's and during my registration process the night before. I responded through tears of sadness, remorse, shame, and self-recrimination, but the element of fear that pervaded the previous four days in Reiss 2 vanished. It occurred to me that this incessant repetition of questions represented the same tactic employed by detectives probing for the truth from the prime suspect in a murder investigation. Paradoxically, I was at once the murderer and the victim. Fortunately, this interrogation occurred at a brightly lit, comfortable conference room table rather than in a chair under a glaring bare light bulb dangling overhead. I didn't need to request a lawyer either—a social worker and a one-on-one psychiatrist were assigned to my case following this initial assessment of my condition. My confidence settled in when I realized I had a dedicated team who would work with and for me every day I remained there.

Because I arrived on a Friday, I had the weekend to settle in. Although we were expected to attend group therapy sessions throughout the day, visiting hours were extended and the atmosphere on Saturday and Sunday seemed more relaxed. Family members were invited to attend a Saturday morning session designed just for them in an effort to help them understand their loved one's issues and how they could support them. John showed up with his unfailing optimism. I'd only been a patient for less than forty-eight hours and already I felt more secure.

After the family meeting John and I were encouraged to share lunch together in the dining room. I proudly escorted him in as if I were the maître d'.

"There's a table over by the window, let's take that one." I draped my multi-colored shawl on one chair and took his jacket to hold another while we joined the line to get our food.

"Wow, this is really nice, Martha. Have you had an appetite?"

"I've been eating like a horse since I got here," I admitted. "Everything is so fresh and there's such a wonderful variety, I sometimes can't choose and shamelessly ask for a little of each."

My relieved, comfortable disposition suddenly came to a halt when I looked up at one of the servers behind the steam table and noticed a man who used to own a little deli near our house. *Oh my God—it's Frank from the deli. What's he doing here? He can't see me like this. I don't want him, or anyone, to know I'm here. God, I hope he doesn't recognize me.*

My face burned with humiliation. I wanted to disappear with the steam evaporating from the mashed potatoes and gravy he stood ready to plop onto my plate.

He'd been hired as part of the weekend kitchen staff at Silver Hill after he sold his business several months earlier. This "small world" encounter completely unnerved me. The last time Frank saw me I would have been picking up my *New York Times* and a coffee-to-go as a snappy business woman hopping the commuter train to my job in the city. I avoided his eyes, pushing my chin down into my chest in hopes he wouldn't recognize me.

Because John followed me in the serving line with no sense of my need for anonymity, the two men shared a "Hey, how're you doin', nice to see you, we miss you at the deli!" moment as I slinked back to our table in the dining room, happy that we'd chosen one so far away from the buffet. My appetite had vanished and my plate remained empty. I felt ashamed, exposed, and utterly humiliated to have someone from my real world see me as a patient in a mental hospital. Suddenly my two planets collided. I realized I would have to begin to cope with explaining myself to the outside world. Suddenly the outside world looked too real for me. If I couldn't forgive myself for what I had done, how could I possibly expect anyone else to understand?

When he set his plate down and took a seat, John picked up on my sudden mood shift.

"What's wrong, honey? You didn't take any lunch."

"I know, I just got a little freaked when I saw Frank. I can't imagine what he must think of me. I wonder if he recognized me."

"Sweetie, even if he did, I honestly don't think he's worrying about it—he probably sees a lot of people here from outside."

"But I just didn't expect to ever see anyone I know here. What if he starts telling people?" It was an absurd thought considering our social circles never overlapped, but nevertheless, I started spiraling into outlandish machinations of the entire state of Connecticut knowing I was an inmate at Silver Hill.

"It doesn't matter who knows, Martha. What matters is you're here and you're going to get well. So let's get you something to eat."

I took a deep breath and quickly glanced over at Frank. He was busy replenishing the steam tray with a pan piled high with mixed vegetables. John was right. Frank never looked over at me and probably wouldn't. He had better things to do than keep track of how many former deli customers showed up at Silver Hill.

"Okay. There's plenty of good stuff at the cold fruit and salad bar. I'll help myself."

For the remainder of our lunch together I did my best to stay lighthearted and hide my fears from John about people knowing—knowing I was a psych patient, knowing I wasn't as strong as I always pretended to be, knowing I tried to kill myself. Now I just wanted to hide from everyone.

Later that afternoon, after John went home, I participated in art therapy. I drew a picture with pastel crayons that started out as a brown mountain. The mountain became a cave with a black hole in the center. I drew a patch of dark green in front of the black hole. Arcs of yellow and blue spewed out of the cave as if they were rockets of sky and light. The therapist leading the session asked each of us to comment on our piece. I had nothing to say. I felt as if I was still inside the cave and wouldn't be coming out for a while. Maybe when I did I'd be able to explain the rest of the picture.

~~

My suspicions that dibs on my insurance coverage were what had held me hostage at Saint Vincent's were confirmed on Monday morning. My doctor at Silver Hill informed me that the insurance company challenged the Silver Hill health plan manager to release me within twenty-four hours because I wasn't covered for more than five days in a hospital. We sat privately in one of the little rooms just off the common area where she coaxed me to provide her with some sort of verbal evidence as proof that I required more time in protective care.

"I hate to have to release you so soon," the psychiatrist bemoaned, "but I don't have enough information on you to support keeping you."

"But I just got here—and I'm only beginning to feel better. Aren't I supposed to feel strong before I leave here?"

I didn't want to exaggerate my condition, but at the same time I knew I shouldn't go home without taking some time to press the reset button on my life. I told her I didn't want to leave because I didn't think I could handle anything other than the steady routine Silver Hill afforded me.

I implored her to keep me for a few more days, not only because I was just coming out of the woods from my suicide attempt, but I was also still reeling from the traumatic experience on Reiss 2. Without hesitation she feverishly tapped her recommendation into her laptop notes as I sat in the tiny office silently beginning to seethe. Those three extra, futile, counterproductive days in Reiss 2 had eaten into my pre-approved coverage allotment. She and I both knew I had only begun to regain my footing. It seemed cruel and illogical that suddenly the problem of "How do I get out of here?" reversed itself to "How do I stay?" She assured me she'd do her best to make the case for me. As my mother used to proclaim, "No news is good news!" I didn't hear another word about leaving and I honestly didn't give a damn what the doctor had to put in her notes to convince the insurance company that I needed to stay at Silver Hill.

As grateful as I felt to be able to remain there, I did learn over the next few days about the stigma attached to mental illness. It is unequivocal, particularly when it's mentioned in a business environment. My job's human resources department required medical verification for my two-week hospitalization and extended absence. That meant I had to actually tell people at my job exactly why I was out of work for so long. The social worker at Silver Hill wisely encouraged me to skirt the issue as we were completing the absentee's short-term disability request.

"You don't have to put any details about why you're in the hospital on this form. Just indicate you have a personal illness and we'll sign it for you," she said.

I took her pen and numbly accepted her dictation word for word as I scribbled my story on the paper. I assumed her experience had obviously told her that disclosing mental illness to an employer is a tacit admission of inadequacy, failure, or even worse, potential implosion in the workplace—a definite liability to the company.

Since I still intended to resume my career after I got out of Silver Hill, understating my medical excuse seemed a safer strategy. On the other hand, betraying my personal integrity because of this fabrication nagged at me. The layer of sugarcoating I lathered all over the ugly truth left me feeling fraudulent and sullied. Regardless, as an officially diagnosed mental patient, I knew I had to either start rehearsing an obscure medical condition story or learn to accept and manage my illness without shame. I needed to face the fact that this illness came with severe societal repercussions and none of it was going to go away. I would now have to go through life either as a con artist or learn to live with it with style and grace.

I spent the rest of the week trying to recalibrate my emotions with antidepressants and anti-anxiety medications. I regained a sense of myself during daily meetings led by competent therapists, volunteers sharing their own stories of addiction and affliction, nutrition sessions, creative writing, physical exercise around the grounds of the hospital, and trips to the residents' library where we received self-help literature and websites for support on the outside.

But the interaction with other patients who occupied the same boat as I did helped the most—a boat of sadness, loneliness, hopelessness, and exhaustion. I didn't feel like such a failure after spending time with other successful professionals in my age group. A few patients had actually checked themselves in to the hospital— they didn't put themselves or their family through the drama that I had. They knew they needed help and they were there to get it. I felt great admiration for their courage and conviction to get well.

Silver Hill provided a safe haven for me, a way station where everyone respected our relationships as confidential, limited, and discreet. The balanced mix of males and females, young and old, provided me with a healthy perspective on how vulnerable we all are to mental disorders. The stories shared, the secrets revealed, the compassion extended within the group of residents I encountered during the seven days I spent at Silver Hill will be with me as a permanent reminder that we all share this place of human vulnerability. Not one of us is immune to the possibility of mental dysfunction, regardless of how strong or buttoned up we may think we are.

I used to think the age-old saying "Misery loves company." meant a bad thing. At Silver Hill misery needed company. It's what got me through the experience and helped me begin healing.

5 | Leaning Against a Bent Oak

Emerging from any institution is a butterfly experience.
Some cocoons might feel cozier than others, but there's no mistaking
the difference between being "in there" and "out here."

— Journal Entry

The sun didn't shine the morning I was scheduled to leave Silver Hill on that cold, mid-March day. I had already met with my social worker and resident doctor before breakfast. Once we determined I was good to go, I packed my bag and began the wait for John to pick me up after the school day let out.

Conflicting thoughts and feelings bubbled up in me as I realized I'd be leaving my shelter. I felt happy to be in a safe, controlled, predictable environment, and at the same time anxious to resume life in the real world. My family assuaged my guilt by lovingly tending to me with phone calls, cards, and visits during the week. The staff achieved their primary goal to stabilize me, to get me squared away so I could face the world in better condition than when I arrived. By showing up for meetings and meals, demonstrating my daily personal hygiene, and interacting with others, I proved to them I had come through my crisis and they had done their job.

Other patients who felt unable to leave the cocoon opted for a month-long in-patient regimen of psychotherapy, medications, and group sessions. I didn't have the thousands of dollars the program required. Parts of me envied them, while on the other hand, the sense of monotony and restriction that accompanied long-term psychiatric care already had begun to bore me. I knew the time had arrived for me to shake hands with reality.

I had almost an entire day to sit in limbo while I waited for John to arrive at four o'clock. No group meetings were scheduled that morning. Everyone gathered in the common room around the fireplace while a young volunteer entertained us by playing his guitar and singing. His curly blond hair fell behind his ears and over the nape of his neck in a loosely fastened ponytail. He wore the plaid flannel shirt and baggy blue jeans uniform of a hippie, even though his youthful looks belonged in the genre of *Metallica*.

It almost felt as if he were auditioning for a job at the hospital since the little hootenanny seemed unplanned and spontaneous. He sat on the edge of the stone hearth, looked around at all of us, and asked, "Um, does anyone have a favorite song they want me to play?"

The skeleton-looking girl with the eating disorder raised her hand. "Yes—can you play 'Puff the Magic Dragon'?"

The moment his fingers began plucking the guitar strings I felt my eyes welling up with tears. My chest tightened with fierce resistance to let them flow. The sound of live music felt so tender and real. I wanted to hide my emotions for fear someone would see me breaking down and retract my release papers. How could the simple act of singing touch my heart so deeply? This impromptu gathering was supposed to be a lighthearted diversion for the patients—and there I sat on the verge of another crying jag.

We spent almost an hour immersed in melodies. Looking back on the deep feelings those simple songs evoked, I realize how connected I am to live music, to the intense personal risk one takes with the act of performing in public. It takes guts to put yourself out in front of others, sharing your voice, your art, your private self's uncertainty about your own talent. He wasn't a fabulous musician and his voice was as common as the simple songs he shared, but sitting in the presence of his music reconnected me with my own humanity. This young volunteer shared his gift with a room full of hopeless people searching for their own worth. I longed to know what my gift for others could possibly be. I longed to know what I had to offer that mattered to someone—to anyone.

When he finished playing, I thanked the young man and told him how much his music inspired me. His bear hug silently conveyed how much it meant to him to play for us.

Time in Silver Hill redefined itself for me. An hour seemed like a day, and a day seemed like an hour. I couldn't believe I'd already been there an entire week, yet it seemed a lifetime since the night I entered the Silver Hill cocoon.

The gray morning moved into an even grayer late afternoon. When John finally arrived I had already retrieved my personal belongings that had been locked away with everyone else's forbidden items. One last check of my vitals—blood pressure and temperature—and I was just a final signature on the patient release form away from leaving.

"Hi honey, I'm sorry I'm a little late. Are you ready?" John asked as he came up the stairs. He looked so handsome in his work clothes. I felt proud of his "old school" style to always wear a dress shirt, tie and jacket, rather than the more casual attire the younger teachers sported. He'd been a music teacher for forty-plus-years and maintained a level of professionalism I genuinely admired. Whenever anyone asked me, "What does your husband do," my answer, "He's a teacher!" bordered on boasting.

"You're not late. I needed the time to say goodbye to a few patients and staff folks. But I'm ready to go now."

Just as inauspiciously as I had arrived, I left Silver Hill. It was getting dark when John tucked me into the car. I steeled my mind for the transition from hospital to home, not knowing what to expect from myself, or anyone else for that matter. I hoped it wouldn't be too scary to be alone in the house while he went to work every day. I prayed for courage. I prayed for enough air to simply breathe. I practiced mindfully while John loaded my bag into the back seat—inhale, exhale, inhale, exhale.

We drove without speaking past the stately woods protecting the hospital grounds. I felt as if I had been on another planet since I last sat in our car's passenger seat. So much had happened during that time—the many group meetings, the constant comings and goings of patients, and most of all, the daily struggle of trying to understand my feelings and how I came to land in this bizarre place called "nervous breakdown."

John took us homeward via a route I'd traveled countless times in the past, and yet everything appeared unfamiliar. I felt like a tourist from another country, being driven along roads I'd never seen before. Neither of us spoke. We hadn't been alone together back in the real world since the nightmare began and now we didn't quite know where to pick things up again. The severity of the crisis versus our relief that I was finally coming home vied for first place on our "things to talk about" list. Unfortunately, neither of us had the courage to tackle either subject. Instead, John favored me with gentle assurances that we'd be home soon.

"I'll make a nice fire in the woodstove for you when we get there. It'll warm right up. I changed the sheets on the bed and the laundry's all done. Are you hungry? Do you want to stop and get something for dinner?"

"Thanks, honey. I'm not too hungry. Let's just get there and we'll see how we feel about everything."

I knew he so desperately wanted to have an ordinary conversation. Back to normal, talking about our jobs, what's playing at the movies, how the baseball teams are doing in spring training, and what's for dinner. Back to before I dropped myself down the rabbit hole.

"I called the kids and told them you'd be home tonight. Maybe they'll phone to say hello. Several people have been calling to find out how you're doing."

"What did you tell them?" I asked, not wanting to hear his answer. Shame's sting choked my response.

"I didn't know what to say, to tell you the truth. I wasn't sure what you wanted me to say. I just let them know you were in good hands and that you'd be home soon."

"Thank you for talking to everyone. I don't want too many people to know what really happened, but I'm sure eventually they all will. Just not now, okay? This is all too humiliating for me right now."

John's relief to have me home again contrasted with my fear of returning there. I felt nervous and afraid to walk through our front door. I knew he had to go to work the next day and I worried about being alone. Most of all I feared the darkest of the dark feelings would revisit the raw shell of a woman I had become.

We turned into our driveway. Everything looked the same in the little starter home we had occupied for thirty-three years— the wicker chairs on the front porch where we often sat sipping chilled Chardonnay on summer evenings, the bird feeders hanging nearby providing us with Mother Nature's free entertainment, and the large picture window staring back at me like a single, dark eye peering out from the house's face.

As soon as John stopped the engine, a sense of dread slipped over me. Suddenly I just wanted to stay put in the car, seat belt firmly strapped across my heaving chest. I felt that my insane actions disqualified me from a once-deserved place in our household. I had irrevocably disrupted our lovingly established balance of home-sweet-home. I betrayed everything hearth and home stood for by selfishly discarding my life. Walking through the front door could only mean I accepted my self-imposed indictment, with no plea bargain on the table.

"C'mon, honey, it's cold out here. I'll bring your bag in later."

John stood holding the car door open, waiting to take my hand and walk me toward the house. I felt nothing—no excitement, no relief, no happiness. I entered the front hall, passed through the living room, and went straight to bed.

∿

The morning of my last day at Silver Hill, I had met with my assigned social worker, Chris, to plan my next steps after hospitalization. Tall, pretty, and smartly dressed, her enthusiastic energy complemented her innate compassion for struggling patients like me. She encouraged me to find a strong support system to help me manage my transition from hospital to real world—"a sturdy oak on which to lean," as she poetically put it.

We sat in the same small room where I'd stripped down to my underwear on my first night of orientation with Kathy, the night nurse.

"Do you have a psychiatrist and a therapist at home?"

"No, just my primary care physician," I answered with a tinge of embarrassment. "I don't know any psychiatrists. Do you?"

I hesitated to even admit that I'd been coasting along for so many years with just my regular doctor managing a depression that should have been assigned to a mental health professional years ago. How could I have overlooked the need for a psychiatrist and therapist when I had felt so deeply depressed for all those months turned into years? Why didn't I take better care of myself? The reality of what my next steps required set in, and I could feel the pressure to reorganize my life mounting within me.

"Well, let me see if I can find someone near your home. I think I've heard of a doctor up in your area who's supposed to be pretty good."

"But I'm going back to work in New York so I should find someone in the city."

Already I began glossing over the actuality that I might not be ready to go back to the intense pressures of a job. With a slightly raised, skeptical eyebrow, Chris peered into her laptop and found an Intensive Outpatient Program (IOP) as well as a talk therapist close to the New York apartment.

"I don't have a psychiatrist to recommend in New York, so you should call this one in Connecticut when you need to refill your antidepressant prescription. But get started in the outpatient program and psychotherapy right away. I'm going to contact them for you today before you leave. How's next Monday for your first appointment?"

Suddenly the ball was in my court, and as I tried to review all the notes she handed me on several sheets of release papers, I glazed over, nodded my head as if I understood, all the while struggling to connect the dots.

"You'll meet with the IOP director and after you're evaluated, they'll put you in group meetings that suit your needs. Here's a number for a therapist, too. She's great and even has a website—give her a call and set up a time to meet with her next week, too."

I left the hospital on a Thursday, made it through the first weekend at home peacefully, and on the following Monday John drove me into the city for the introduction to the Intensive Outpatient Program that Chris had set up on my behalf.

～∽

The afternoon sun dramatically illuminated the Hudson River's cold roiling water as we sped along the West Side Highway without the usual rush hour delays. I felt anxious returning to New York, since this highway was a sad reminder of the last time I left the city in the ambulance, in darkness, amid rush hour traffic. It felt unnatural to be driving into Manhattan on a weekday, in the middle of the day, with John—and not going to a job, or at least a job I could relate to.

We arrived on time to a crowded reception room crammed with two large, overstuffed couches and several folding chairs.

A pleasant intake counselor emerged from a hallway and brought me into an even smaller office. She seemed almost too young to handle the task of sorting out my therapy plan. Although her closely cropped green and orange hairdo, theatrical chandelier earrings, and trendy outfit perfectly suited her for the city, I couldn't help but wonder if I'd be better off back in Fairfield County with the rest of the older gals who managed their depression in a more traditional setting.

She opened our meeting with the company line. "We're happy you've chosen the Life Awareness Center for your recovery."

I numbly nodded agreement to her as she situated herself at an empty desk with pen and clipboard. She looked at me with eyes that seemed to say, "What are you doing here? You don't fit the mold of the worn-out drug abusers and anorexics we usually see."

I couldn't blame her. I showed up as a tidy suburbanite wearing a signature pearl necklace to prove it. In contrast to the waiting room filled with teenagers, gnarly old men, and severely weight-challenged women, I looked pretty damn normal. Instead of answering her unspoken question, I self-consciously pulled my sweater up around my collarbone to conceal my incongruous accessory.

The long list of questions she recited now seemed all too familiar. I felt distracted by the furniture in the small, windowless office. It looked as if it had been appropriated from a local flea market. The oversized desk consumed the space, leaving little room for the two mismatched chairs we occupied. An unforgiving, overhead light made me feel exposed and stifled. Bacon and garlicky smells from the ground floor deli permeated the air, taunting my now knotted stomach.

I reprimanded myself as if I were a child. *Okay, Martha, this is supposed to be good for you and you're going to have to get over what the place looks like. Stay open-minded and supportable. You need help. You, for one, should know better than to assume that what you see is what you get. Particularly since you've managed to fool so many people for so long about yourself.*

After a brief interview with the intake counselor and a longer wait in the reception area, the program director came out and handed me a schedule with three-times-a-week group therapy sessions. "Living in Sobriety," "Understanding Alcohol and Sobriety/Women," and "Relapse Recovery." Seven-thirty PM, Tuesday, Wednesday, Thursday—bing, bang, boom.

I paused and reviewed my new life's agenda. Wait a minute. How come these are all about alcohol and sobriety? No groups for the depths of depression and attempted suicide? No group named "Understanding and Dealing With Fuck-It-All-Anyway"?

I refrained from jumping to any negative conclusions and took the appointment sheet without questioning the nature of the groups, assuring the counselor I'd be there the next day for my first session of "Living in Sobriety," reassuring myself I would find my way in this new and foreign world of rehab.

The good news was at least I didn't have to schlep around the city to get myself back on track. The talk therapist my social worker recommended had her office right around the corner from the outpatient clinic. The apartment, rehab, and therapist all located in one convenient neighborhood. One-stop shopping. The proverbial ducks were lining up. I began to feel my life coming back in alignment. I prayed the planets would position themselves in my favor as well.

∞

I spent my first week out of the hospital sleeping at home but driving into New York for Intensive Outpatient sessions on Tuesday, Wednesday, and Thursday. Instead of traveling the sixty-five miles to a city job as I had done all those years, I now commuted to my new occupation—healing my broken spirit.

My plan to knit work life neatly together with rehabilitation took shape when miraculously, and quite prematurely, I returned to work in New York the next week. I figured since I would be in the city anyway for my outpatient sessions, I might as well get myself back in the saddle at work.

The following Monday morning, I stood on the train platform and gripped the valise filled with fresh clothes I would need for the week while I stayed overnight at the apartment. It felt as if a bizarre lifetime had transpired since I'd last boarded my usual 7:09 Metro North train. Loved ones urged me to take more time before I jumped back into the rigors of living the dual life of Country Mouse/City Mouse, but I rationalized the necessity of returning to normal life by pumping myself up with pseudo-confidence.

I've got to get back to work because I need something to do. I've got to make sure nothing falls between the cracks with all the client projects that are happening. I haven't spoken with anyone there to see how things are going. I bet the place is falling apart without me.

I convinced myself working was a way to reclaim my spirit, still under the delusion that this depression was strictly psychological and had nothing to do with any physical incapacity. I intended to suck it up, shield my pride, and act as if nothing had happened.

The stark memory of a crowded elevator ride the first day I returned to work has proved to me just how devious I became in the cover-up.

As we all squeezed ourselves into the cramped cage along with several other co-workers, a friendly guy from the finance department asked, "Hey, Martha. Haven't seen you for a while. Heard you were in the hospital. You okay?"

"Hi there, uh, yeah, sure. I've been out for a few weeks. Had a little heart issue. I'm fine now. But thanks for asking," I muttered.

My face flushed with intense embarrassment as I felt the effect my alibi had on the now-attentive listeners sharing the interminable ascent to the twenty-first floor. Another co-worker instantly averted my glance. I felt exposed—convinced everyone knew I was lying, as if my secret bled like a stab wound through the front of my light blue business suit and revealed the raw truth of my crazy condition.

I raised my eyes to check if Mr. Finance bought my fib. He seemed satisfied knowing I'd survived a heart problem. He didn't press me for any gory details, and I felt grateful for that concession.

Another colleague averted her glance while the deafening silence in the tiny space consumed what little air remained for me to suck in. I felt sure she must have known the truth, even though her thumb nervously tapping against her purse's shoulder strap told me she was probably worried about being late for a meeting. When the elevator door finally released me, I bolted to my corner office, closed the door, and did my best to swallow the bitter pill of deceit. I couldn't tell which felt worse: lying to others or lying to myself about my mental illness.

My staff greeted me with a mixed bag of relief, concern, and overall enthusiasm. I felt happy to be missed, but within a few hours my energy level was somewhere down at the level of the city subway system. Returning to work was a big mistake. Although my game face came in mighty handy, the focus and mental fortitude necessary to get through the day eluded me, not to mention the lingering effects of what I call "game face hangover." The amount of energy necessary to maintain a consistent look and feel of unfettered, neatly disguised normalcy utterly exhausted me—something akin to the drained feeling that accompanies the morning after an evening with more than a few martinis.

∿∾

By the time I got to the apartment that evening, feelings of self-doubt greeted me at the door. Had I returned to work too soon? Shouldn't I have at least stayed a week or two out in Connecticut to regain my footing? Did I really think my job would suffer if I took more time off?

The first floor, studio apartment I had grown to love now felt unfamiliar and unwelcoming. The four walls that used to be my little hideaway now held my secret. They stood as witnesses to the night I gave up on life. I felt embarrassed in their presence. When I noticed the large, outspread handprints on the back windows overlooking the garden, my heart sank. My sister had told me the emergency rescue team went through the adjoining apartment's front door to gain access to the common back yard area both units shared. Their mutton-sized hands, shockingly visible on the sooty glass pane, gave tacit testimony as to how hard they tried to find a way to get to me. They ultimately came through the back door. Now, safely returned to the scene of the crime, I felt mortified at the thought of what I had done and to what extent total strangers went through as they scrambled to save me.

I immediately switched on the television set for distraction with the nightly news. My usual pour of the self-medicating wine or vodka that kept me company every night was no longer an option, now that I was assigned to the ranks of rehabilitating substance abusers. The truth was, I didn't even miss it. The knowledge that alcohol had left me so vulnerable to self-destruction placed a huge barrier between me and the bottle. I knew I'd feel scared if someone set even a glass of wine in front of me—not for fear of the desire to actually drink it, but remembering the horrible feeling of what it allowed me to do to myself just a few weeks before was too much to bear.

~∽

In spite of my effort to prove my commitment to the agency, two weeks after returning to work I lost my job. The director of human resources came to my office to inform me my position had been eliminated. Organizational restructuring is how they couched it. As a professional, I tried to accept that the faltering economy determined my fate. I had no proof that my illness contributed to my sudden and unexpected joblessness. My disgrace about what I'd done and the stigma of my depression diagnosis made me wonder if they had seen through my veiled excuse on the extended absence form from Silver Hill Hospital.

I couldn't get the human resources director who delivered the bad news to level with me. Was it really restructuring, or did my absence have anything to do with the decision? We both acknowledged I recently scored the highest achievable agency ranking on my performance review. I couldn't imagine why my name should be on the cut list and desperately needed an answer.

"No, no—it's a business decision the agency has made. It

has nothing to do with illness or poor performance," Mr. HR Hatchetman stammered in defense. I wanted to believe him, but my world had turned so upside down, this edict felt inhumane. My job was my life, and in the past few weeks my life was at stake. There's rehab for alcoholics, but where's the rehab for workaholics, I wondered.

The HR guy left me alone and I packed up my office. In the cab ride back to the apartment, I fiercely debated with myself about whether I could make it to my scheduled group therapy session at the Life Awareness Center. I muffled an outburst to myself through indignant tears. "Screw it—screw it all. There's no point to any of this crap." I caught the cab driver's concern as he eyed me in his rearview mirror, probably wondering if my tears would cost him his tip. When he dropped me off at my building, I gave him an extra buck. He nodded a thank you, and as he stuffed the fare into his wallet I gathered all my bags overflowing with ex-office stuff out onto the curb. I looked up and noticed the taxi hadn't raced away. The driver rolled down his window and peered out at me.

"You be okay, ladeee. You look like nice person."

He smiled sympathetically and drove away in search of his next fare.

I sighed and wished I'd given him a fatter tip.

When I opened the door to the empty studio apartment, it suddenly seemed enormous, dark and still—no longer the welcoming haven I so depended on after a long day's work. How did my cozy cocoon become such a scary cave? In my heart I knew the answer. This adorable little apartment had been violated. My unconscionable actions had insulted it, dirtied it, spoiled it, and robbed it of what it had always offered me—peace and relaxation. I felt ashamed, as if I had cheated on a lover or lied to a child.

I turned on the television, although that night I didn't care one bit about the world's news. I just needed the sound to fill the space, since Merlot and Stolichnaya had also been fired from their job of keeping me company. The voice inside my head chided me for buckling under the avalanche of bad news about my unemployment. I sat down on the edge of the bed, dazed, wondering what I should do next.

I can't call John. This'll just be one more thing for him to worry about. Who should I call? What should I do? Maybe I should have taken the train home to Connecticut instead of coming to the apartment.

My trusty motto, "Just proceed," dug itself out from under the rubble of emotions and confusion. It refused to be ignored.

Just as I had dragged myself to work every day for all those years, I knew I had to get myself out the door, only a few city blocks down the street, and into that evening's group meeting at the Life Awareness Center. My mind put up a fierce argument nevertheless.

But I don't want to go. It won't matter anyway. Nothing matters. Besides, it's a new group and they don't know me, so what's the difference?

I sat on the edge of the bed watching the clock, anxious as the minutes passed while I wrestled with my choice. *Should I try to make it to the meeting? I'll probably be late and I hate being late for anything.* I wondered if being late was enough of an excuse to bail on the idea and end the whole debate.

In an instant I realized my hopeless, jobless life depended on this decision. I grabbed my purse and jacket, and checked my face for smudged mascara from my weepy cab ride.

"Just proceed. Yeah, just proceed—and while you're at it, go kick ass somewhere!" I shouted as I slammed the apartment door behind me.

The miserable day of losing my job ended with the challenge of joining a new group at the rehab center. After sitting through the previous two nights of my first week in IOP, I asked my caseworker to replace one of my alcohol abuse sessions with one that focused more on depression-related issues. I thought it might round out my rehab repertoire. Unfortunately, that night I couldn't have been more disinterested in meeting anyone—

anywhere—on Planet Earth, especially the people with whom I was about to share the next couple of hours.

I showed up in the lobby area almost on time.

"Hi, I'm Martha Rhodes and I've been reassigned to tonight's 'Women's Issues' meeting."

"It's already started, but you can go in if you're quiet." The receptionist waved a long index finger over her shoulder without looking up from her computer screen. "They're in room four."

I could barely see the faded "4" on the closed door as I made my way down the dimly lit hall. I hesitated for a second, giving myself one last mental kick in the ass as I slipped through the sliver of space between the door frame into the packed room.

The group leader summoned everyone's attention. Her six-inch-high, intricately constructed hairdo framed her dark complexion as she commanded the room like a queenly mother gathering her court. She sat on the edge of a black leather swivel chair at the far end of the room. Her crossed leg naturally projected her right foot out toward the center of the room, showing off an unusually high, high-heeled shoe. I imagined that standing, she'd measure well over six feet tall, thanks to her extreme coiffeur and footwear. Her expressive eyes directed me to take the last available seat.

Adding to the still stinging mortification of being fired, my late arrival drew everyone's attention toward me. I felt acutely out of place in this windowless, stuffy room—as if I'd shown up at a nudist colony in a snowsuit. I maneuvered myself into a nattily upholstered chair crammed in between an assemblage of people, the likes of whom I had never encountered.

My mind scrambled with critical curiosity as I eyed the perfectly coiffed transvestite—dressed in a polyester corporate-style suit resurrected from the eighties—sitting demurely across the overcrowded room. An obese, profusely tattooed teenager reeking of sour attitude wedged herself in the corner. A petite, nervous young woman sitting next to the group leader uncontrollably picked at invisible scabs on her bared arms, neck, and shoulders, and a nearly toothless, withered older woman in a baggy powder blue jogging suit shared the right armrest of my chair.

What the hell am I doing in a place like this? I'm not like these people. I'm NOT!! I have a normal home with a normal husband and normal children. These people are from another world—certainly not mine.

Keisha, the group leader, officially opened the meeting.

"Okay, let's get started by each of you introducing yourself—first name only—and briefly tell us why you're here. Then I'll hand out an exercise sheet we'll all do together and we'll end with our commitments for the next week."

She referred to the roster of names resting in her lap as she prepared to take attendance.

"Marlene, since you've been here the longest, why don't you start us out."

Now, how is she ever going to be able to use that pen she's holding with those inch-long fingernails, and how did she get those little diamonds to stick on her pinkies?

We went around the room with our introductions, mine being last. When my turn finally came I could hardly breathe, much less state my name and reason for being there.

"Hello, my name is Martha and I'm here because of depression." Taking a pause I mumbled, "Oh yeah, uh, and I lost my job today, too."

After three heartbeats of silence, the entire room gasped with what felt like surprise, disbelief, heart-felt sympathy—I couldn't tell which. Instantly a round of boisterous applause erupted as everyone congratulated me for making it to the meeting despite my bad day. The older woman without teeth sitting next to me took my hand in hers and squeezed it compassionately. My tears streamed, unstoppable and hot, not because I felt sorry for myself—I'd taken care of that self-indulgence earlier in the cab ride. Rather, my heart literally cracked wide open with the purest shot of *simpatico* and gratitude for a group of strangers I had only moments before judged to be inferior to, of all people, me—pathetic, rudderless, self-righteous me.

This scenario determined my moment of ultimate surrender. Surrendering to the not-knowing-what's-next, to the anything-can-happen and it's-all-happening-for-a-reason thinking. I knew my life was now redefined in terms of "Before" and "After" my deranged detour. The members of the therapy group unknowingly became my tour guides as I wended my way through rehab's unfamiliar territory.

Magically, I began to breathe more easily as my heart stopped pounding. The judge and jury exited the courtroom inside my head, enabling me to listen to each person's story with genuine empathy. Stories of lifelong despair over an abducted child, relationships annihilated by alcohol abuse and persistent violence, jobs forfeited and careers destroyed in favor of drug addiction. Everyone fighting her demons while holding on to life with white knuckles. The common denominator of our mutual humanity bound us as if we'd known each other for a lifetime.

What mystified me most, however, was how everyone in the room managed to laugh at herself in one way or another. For all their serious dilemmas, they still succeeded in finding a kernel of humor or irony in them. Did they hold a secret I had yet to discover? Did I take myself too seriously, and did I need to invent a new way to hold my joy and my sadness, my wins and my losses?

When the session adjourned an hour and a half later, I descended to the street in the packed elevator with several of the women, our butts and shoulders unapologetically touching. We shared "good-byes," "see-ya-next-weeks," and "take care of yourself" as I strolled across town to the apartment I'd resisted leaving a couple of hours earlier. My mind swirled with questions about what to do next, but my heart heaved with relief. I had found—at least temporarily—a placeholder for my interrupted life.

∿∾

During the first few weeks of outpatient therapy I continued to stay in the Manhattan apartment with vain hopes of finding another job. Without honestly acknowledging it, however, my new occupation became Tuesday visits to the New York talk therapist set up by Silver Hill, and attending the three-days-a-week group sessions at the Life Awareness Center that were primarily designed to handle addictions.

Every meeting opened with each person's first-name introduction, followed by "and I'm a drug addict" or "and I'm an alcoholic." More men than women attended the groups. Many of them were crawling their way back to earning rights to their child's custody or at the very least, unsupervised visitation.

We usually took the same seat in the room every meeting. My spot was third chair from the door on the right hand side, next to a burly bear of a guy named Jason.

"I've done everything the judge ordered," he opened. "I got a steady job, I go to AA meetings every day, I send the money every two weeks when I get paid. She's already got the house and the car which I can't drive anyway cuz of my DUI. And I'm sober eighteen months now—damn, my pee is so god-damn clean I could drink it myself! But I still can't just stop by and hold my kid. She always says he's busy and I shouldn't come."

I could hear Jason's frustration when his voice cracked. Worse than that, I felt his grief, his utter remorse as he extended his trembling hands out in front of himself pleading to the gods of forgiveness to please explain what else he had to do to regain his life. His entire body in the chair next to me emanated palpable contrition. My heart broke for him.

Other men chimed in, bemoaning the unfairness of their wives, ex- and otherwise, who took them to court for their drunken behavior and drug addictions, and who used the kids as retaliatory leverage. Lots of DUI's hung their heads in shame while doing their rehab time to regain a driver's license, and a couple of beat-looking old guys augmented their Alcohol Anonymous meetings with these group therapy discussions. There were even a couple of convicted drug addicts fulfilling probation requirements.

They seemed like decent fellows and it was hard for me to imagine them as anything but devoted, loving fathers, sons, brothers, and husbands based on their intensely expressed commitment to overcome their demons.

One spunky gal didn't have much to share about her professed drug and food addictions that she'd overcome two decades earlier, but she knew everyone there and they treated her almost like a sister. She seemed perfectly normal. I didn't understand why she needed to be there until I realized this was her world, a place that afforded her a sense of belonging and guaranteed her sobriety.

The only other woman in the group was about my age and appeared to come from money. Her perfectly styled hair, makeup, jewelry, and clothing hinted of Upper East Side, or maybe even a Fifth Avenue penthouse. Like myself, she spoke quietly and withheld most of her story, other than the fact that she could no longer keep even a bottle of cooking wine in her kitchen because she'd drink it by lunchtime.

Even though I tried, I failed to make the same connection for myself. I operated from the experience of surviving suicide, and although alcohol ferried me across the river of doom, I felt isolated and misunderstood among the alkies and druggies—like the odd man out—whenever I self-consciously mumbled my introductory tag line, "and I tried to kill myself." No one else's story resembled mine. No one ever talked about hopelessness and despair or waking up every morning wishing they were dead, although I think it's safe to say they probably did.

My persistent feelings of detachment from the group prompted me to reassess my own reasons for showing up at the meetings. I had never thought of myself as a bona fide alcoholic. College drinking and early-married life didn't allow it for want of "fun money." Wine or Scotch on the weekends and a perfunctory cocktail at a business dinner summed up the beginnings of my official, routine drinking career sometime during my late thirties.

The first prescription of antidepressants from my original psychiatrist in my mid-forties did not come with his cautioning me, "Do not drink alcohol when taking this medication." We never discussed my drinking at that time. We were too busy sorting out the damages done to my psyche from childhood molestation. I had plenty of excess baggage to share with that first doctor that didn't involve drinking issues. I took the Zoloft he prescribed each month and spent a couple of years pouring my guts out to him about my childhood upbringing, my current relationship with my own children, and how I needed a way to cope with life in general. Eventually I felt I could manage with the new perspectives I gained through his counsel and the ongoing, gradually increasing dose of medicine.

Over the decades of ever-present job stress and diminishing return on the antidepressants, however, alcohol became my go-to pacifier. Alcohol made me feel better or, more accurately, feel nothing. The pain of living dulled with every sip, and in my progressive depressed state, that pain rivaled just about any other daily discomfort. I never correlated my diagnosis of depression with alcohol, especially since I had my morning pill of good mood medicine to cover that problem. Little did I know that as the antidepressant decreased in its effectiveness, my consumption of liquor increased. I unconsciously self-medicated myself every time I poured a drink. I created what ended up as a perfect storm that destroyed me in every way—physically, emotionally, and mentally.

Looking back, a health professional friend told me that my eventual excessive drinking categorized me as a secondary alcoholic, with a primary depression. Based on the miserable condition I was in at the time I struggled with attending IOP and—regardless of what bucket of illness I ultimately fell into—any shape, manner, or form of group therapy meeting did provide me with some benefit, directly or indirectly.

I didn't openly question why I landed in substance abuse

meetings instead of hunkering down with a group of kindred spirits hell-bent on exterminating themselves. But I unconsciously longed for more understanding about the mysterious suicide thoughts lurking in my heart. I'd leave a meeting with a festering frustration and ask myself, "Why doesn't anyone want to talk about killing themselves in these meetings? Why don't they either share their own experience with suicide or help me get a grip on why I did what I did?"

I felt I had no choice but to trust my health care providers' opinions that I belonged in the ranks of the addicted, so I dutifully showed up every week—on time and according to the schedule.

∽∾

At first the routine mandatory pee in the cup before every group meeting proving one's abstinence from drugs and alcohol filled me with indignation. I knew drugs and alcohol (at this point) were the furthest things from my heart's desire. Booze and I had met our Waterloo the night I mixed it with the Xanax, and my terror of it squelched any penchant for even a sip. Eventually I came to realize, however, that I was in a pool of people whose successful rehabilitative process depended on this particular "show and tell" exercise.

I actually got pretty adept at maneuvering myself in the tiny bathroom stall to deposit my urine sample in the little plastic container, sans drips. Once filled, a tight screw-on lid secured its contents, which went into a sealed bag with my name, date, and time recorded on the accompanying laboratory form. I never did get over the minor embarrassment of subsequently appearing in the meeting room in front of twelve strangers, clear plastic bag in hand with my brilliant yellow urine in full view. But once I placed it on top of the pile along with everyone else's proof of purity awaiting the judiciary lab pick-up, I unruffled my feathers and settled in for the real work to be done in that evening's session.

∽∾

After ten weeks of Intensive Outpatient therapy, I relaxed my resistance to group therapy and acknowledged to myself and to others my genuine appreciation for the Life Awareness Center. The support, education, and accountability greatly benefited me. I began to feel part of life again, albeit a new and different life. I grew to appreciate the group members with a newfound wisdom and unbounded empathy. The mutual pain and life struggle brought us to common ground on which to stand and deliver the commitments necessary to redefining ourselves and reshaping our lives.

I still hadn't figured out how I fit into this world of rehabilitation, however. Would my life now be defined as "former alcoholic" or "sober"? Could I trust that abstaining from liquor would guarantee me safe passage to my future? Or would I still be battling the demons that incessantly whispered in my ear every day, "What's the point of living? Why bother with anything? Nothing matters anyway." Those thoughts—not the bottle—haunted me relentlessly. I knew I could easily choose not to drink, but my fear of living outweighed my fear of dying.

I felt convinced that my membership dues belonged to the Crazies Club. My affliction wasn't dependence on cocaine, weed, or Johnny Walker—my problems existed because I had tried to kill myself; because I didn't see any point to living a life filled with so much random hopelessness—a life where even the slightest reminder of something in my past sent me into an abyss of regret and self-recrimination.

This hopelessness was as visceral and real to me as the sun rising and the moon setting every twenty-four hours. No amount of alcohol or drugs would stave it off. Death continued to be a fascination; romancing the past only fed the melancholy and thwarted any sense of a bright future. I frequently dreamed of people who had died, some of whom I thought I'd forgotten. Others' painful absence, like my deceased parents', duly served to fuel my sense of isolation. I longed to be with the deceased and inhabit their world instead of the one I felt trapped in. It all boiled down to one nagging question: "What is the point of all this?"

I wanted to understand what kind of adversary my depression really was: saboteur, provocateur, disabler, dominator. I had to know if I would ever be out of harm's way. Feeling like a hostage in a middle ground, all I saw was the sad, scary, regretful past with no vision, no concept whatsoever for the future. I longed for a fairy godmother with a magic wand to come and transform my world and me in it. I had already tried crying "Uncle!" and failed.

During the following few weeks of IOP and appointments with a New York psychotherapist, I nurtured a false hope that I would soon find another job and jump back on the advertising treadmill. I refreshed my resume and made a few calls to former colleagues and a couple of executive recruiters, but most of the time I felt like a shiny chrome ball banging around the tilted, noisy surface of a pinball machine. I didn't know who had their hands on the flipper handles, but I lived with the constant anxiety that someone other than myself was calling the shots. I fretted about slipping into one of the machine's holes with bells chiming and lights a-blinking, as I disappeared down the chute—game over.

The eight-week program at the Life Awareness Center came to a close based on the insurance company's pre-approval statement. Living in two places seemed like an unnecessary expense, and since no new job appeared, I worried about money constantly. Spring delivered daffodils and longer, warmer days, and the weekends I spent at home in Connecticut with John felt more comfortable and supportive than living alone in the apartment where I holed myself up like a cave dweller. The time had arrived for me to rejoin the world for no other reason than to simply know I could do it—to live in spite of myself.

Early on a Monday morning in May I packed my usual city bag and started out the front door to catch the train to New York. The air felt cool and clear as the sun introduced itself through the dewy leaves on the magnolia tree in the front yard. The birds had arrived at the feeders and quarreled with each other for a breakfast perch. Suddenly, I put down my bag and took a seat in the wicker rocking chair on the front porch. I heard the train's engine echoing through the woods as it approached the station half a mile down the road. I sat paralyzed as I envisioned the commuters springing from their parked cars, balancing coffee cups, newspapers, and briefcases as they dashed up the platform stairs before the train doors slammed shut. I listened for the two short "toot's" the train always made to signal its departure. The engine rumbled loudly as it first accelerated, but soon softened to a distant rumble the further it traveled down the tracks.

I fought to quiet the inner voice that rudely insisted I had failed at my job, failed at my career, and failed at my life. I closed my eyes and tried to convince myself that not getting on the train that morning wasn't cowardice and that I hadn't chickened out.

The truth is, I didn't actually decide to move out of the apartment and back to Connecticut that day. The morning air, the magnolia tree, the birds, and the rocking chair on the front porch formed a committee and made the decision for me. They all knew I'd have a better chance of surrendering to life—as life chose to serve itself up to me—at home where I belonged.

6 | MEDICATION MERRY-GO-ROUND

*"If you drink much from a bottle marked 'poison' it is certain
to disagree with you sooner or later."*

– Lewis Carroll, *Alice in Wonderland*

A month had passed when I noticed the nearly empty bottle of
EffexorXR prescribed by the hospital. The psychotherapist
couldn't write me a refill prescription, nor could anyone at the
Life Awareness Center. Fortunately, I remembered the name of
the Connecticut psychiatrist that the Silver Hill social worker
recommended. He could give me my monthly supply of meds. At
first I hesitated to call him because I clung to the idea that I would
quickly find another job in New York, as I had always done in the
past. I planned to find a mid-town doctor I could conveniently fit
into a lunch hour. Now that I was officially out of the apartment,
I had no choice but to find a doctor close to home.

Leaving the city and acknowledging what felt like defeat was,
in itself, a bitter pill to swallow. Ironically, it was only the beginning
of what I've come to regard as the Medication Merry-Go-Round.

∿

Almost twenty years earlier—long before the actual suicide
attempt and just after my fantasy about jumping in front of that
New York crosstown bus—the first psychiatrist I'd ever consulted
prescribed Zoloft as a way to manage my depression. I was in
my early forties and immersed in raising a family while working
fourteen-hour days. I had vaguely heard of antidepressants from
a fellow colleague who herself buckled under the ad world's

pressures, but I had no personal knowledge of depression as an actual illness. I regarded it as a vague emotional condition that women used as a catchall complaint to sum up their lives when things didn't go as they had planned.

Back then I'd seen a talk therapist a few years earlier to deal with nagging remnants of childhood issues. I wasn't officially diagnosed with depression, nor was any prescription written to assuage my dark moods. I had never been to a licensed psychiatrist until a friend in my women's support group recommended one when we all realized I was losing my grip. I took the first name offered and called Dr. H, who practiced out of his house nestled in the wooded area of a nearby town in Connecticut.

I arrived on a gray Saturday morning and as he had instructed me to do during our introductory telephone call, I opened a door marked "Office" and let myself into a little foyer connecting the main house with his psychiatric practice. I poked my head around a half-opened door to an adjoining room where I assumed we'd be meeting, wondering if he had heard my car tires disturb the driveway's gravel. I hoped the front door I intentionally pulled shut as loudly as I could had sufficiently announced my presence in the silent, empty space.

The dark pine paneling drew minimal light from the one small window at the room's end. A low-beamed ceiling and plush carpeting on the floor created an insulated yet cozy atmosphere. I stood in the middle of the room, unsure if I should call out a "Helloooooo?" or just wait in the deafening stillness that fed my growing apprehension. I wasn't sure what to expect from a psychiatrist, and I was even more dubious as to what I should say or do. My inexperienced Hollywood version involved lying on a couch, staring into space and responding to cryptic questions with revealing answers I conjured from the depths of my tortured soul. Since I didn't see a couch, my scene already needed editing.

I adjusted myself in the deep seat of a well-worn upholstered chair—poised to meet my new sanity savior—when a heavy wooden pocket door slid to one side and Dr. H almost magically emerged. He was much older than I'd expected. His thinning, colorless hair seemed desperate to find a comfortable position on his head. Thick, black-rimmed glasses and a bulbous nose gave him the look of an absent-minded professor. A bushy mustache concealed his mouth so that when he spoke, its sporadic movement distracted me from his words.

He greeted me with a welcoming but formal demeanor. I extended my hand too late to catch his before he took his position in an authoritatively positioned armchair.

"Mrs. Rhodes, please sit back and make yourself comfortable. I'll begin with a few questions and then perhaps you'll have some questions for me."

After listening for thirty minutes to my complaints of sleep disturbance, chronic sadness, job stress, hopelessness, and an inordinate preoccupation with death and dying, he asked, "And how long have you been experiencing these symptoms?"

Suddenly my litany of complaints came to a screeching halt. It seemed almost a minute before the sorriest truth came to light. I lowered my head into my chest and covered my face with both hands.

"Doctor, I can't tell you how long I've felt so sad. All I know is, I cannot remember the last time I actually felt happy."

Dr. H came up with a diagnosis as simply as if he'd picked an apple from the lowest branch on a tree.

"You have clinical depression," he stated flatly.

"Okay, you're right—I feel very depressed. But what does that mean in terms of how I'm going to get to work every day without falling apart?"

"Do you have a computer?" (Remember, this was in the early 1990s.)

"Yes, I've got one at work and I'm still trying to figure out how to use it," I replied, almost embarrassed to admit my technical incompetence.

"Have you ever had your computer freeze up on you? Where the cursor on the monitor screen won't move and none of the keys on the keyboard respond when you press them?"

"Actually, that happened to me the other day and I had to get the Help Desk to come."

"Your brain is like a computer," Dr. H explained. "When you've got too many programs open, your computer's processor can't always handle what you're asking it to do, because you've got too many operations trying to push through it."

I've always related to analogies, so his next explanation instantly lit the invisible light bulb hovering above my head.

"Right now your brain is in overload and it doesn't have the capacity to process all that you need to feel happy. I'm going to give you a medicine that will help your brain function as it should. We'll start you on a low dose and see how you feel in two weeks."

The prescription for Zoloft seemed to help initially. The preoccupation with death and dead people that had driven me to schedule my first appointment with him miraculously vanished. Zoloft erased my need to constantly suppress an impending crying jag. Part of the feel-good bargain accompanying this medication, however, was emotional numbness, lack of libido, and weight gain which he neglected to warn me about. It wasn't until I'd replaced most of my wardrobe's skirts and slacks with a size larger that I brought it to his attention a couple of months later.

"Oh, yes, you're gaining a little weight because of the meds. Try to watch your caloric intake." At the time, I simply nodded and vowed to cut out anything fattening. I regarded these side effects as fleeting and in keeping with the breakneck pace of the rest of my life. The up side of the deal panned out favorably. A heavier body didn't seem to matter given how much lighter my mood felt.

With restored energy and confidence thanks to the Zoloft, my career took off when I won a senior level position at one of New York's largest, most prestigious advertising agencies. The agency was so big it maintained an infirmary and full-time nurse. As a newly appointed senior partner, I underwent a required physical assessment with Nurse Patty.

"Your blood pressure and heart rate are terrific, Martha."

"Thanks. I'm probably one of the healthiest people on the planet. I rarely get sick and I'm very lucky that good health runs in my family." I touted all this fully intending to assure Nurse Patty that the agency had indeed made an excellent choice when they hired me. They'd never have to worry about too many sick days with me on the job.

"Good—great to hear that. Are you on any medications?"

"Uh, no, not really. Just the usual Tylenol for the occasional headache." I lied right through my healthy-as-a-horse teeth.

The common—and negative—attitude about depression at that time had already seeped into my psyche. Depression was regarded as a failing, a breakdown of a person's spirit, having nothing to do with physical disability. I didn't want this major advancement in my career jeopardized in any way, so I checked with a friend and former human resources director at my previous agency about how to handle the impending examination.

"Absolutely do not tell anyone you're on antidepressants. They don't have to know this and you are not obligated to tell them." She adamantly drew the line for me between personal and professional medical information. I felt relieved for her input, but the seed of secrecy we planted in that conversation flourished into a patch of weeds as I constantly guarded my condition and its medication for many years afterward. No one other than my husband had the slightest clue that I got up every morning and dropped a depression drug. In retrospect, living as a closeted depressed person took more energy than it was probably worth. Living a lie is in itself very depressing.

In those earlier career days I didn't have the apartment in the city, and the fourteen- to sixteen-hour workdays included a two-and-a-half-hour (one-way) commute that even I couldn't believe

I tolerated. But taking the antidepressant kept me on track, kept me even-tempered, kept me from feeling sad and self-defeating. John's comments of how much better I seemed made everything, including the side effects, worth the price of admission. The antidepressant not only relieved my unpredictable mood swings, it soothed his nerves as well.

Zoloft did the trick for several years afterward. That is, until the dosage gradually crept up to the maximum and I still didn't feel normal. I felt as if a gauzy sheet of film separated me from the rest of the world. When I attended the funeral of a dear friend and couldn't shed a single tear, I began to question if I was even human anymore. When anything joyful occurred, my reaction fell far short of celebratory.

Rather than switch to a different medication, I decided that the ever-present numbness rendered my life as boring. I missed having a good, healthy cry every now and then. I longed to feel a little pull in my heart when I'd see one of those feel-good-human-interest stories on the evening news. My point of view on anything became one big "Whatever…"

"Want to go to the movies tonight?"

"Whatever…"

"You're promoted to vice president—congratulations!"

"Whatever…"

"Mad Cow Disease is spreading all over Europe!!"

"Whatever…"

The dilemma: do I continue to feel uninterested and uninteresting, or can I live with the pervasive sadness?

I went with the latter option. I gave up the expensive psychiatrist and took myself off Zoloft for several months, hoping I could live without the meds. My little experiment failed miserably. Within three months I started falling apart again, unable to cope with work and home life without some form of psychopharmacological life raft.

Six months after I eliminated the Zoloft, I showed up at

a new primary care physician's office in a swamp of tears and hopelessness. My sister had recommended her.

"Dr. T is new to the area and although she's a general practitioner, she really gets it about women," my sister said. "She's been prescribing an antidepressant for me and I feel much better. And she'll make sure you get your Pap smear and mammograms, too. Give her a call and let her know I sent you."

I rarely went to a doctor since I had such great general health, so having a one-stop-shop physician made perfect sense to me. I was pleased to get an appointment within a few days. Her small private office felt comfortable and user-friendly. When Dr. T walked in for our first visit wearing handsome leather boots, a stylish long skirt, and flowing tunic sweater, I could easily have mistaken her for an artist rather than a doctor. Her mane of auburn hair framed a flawless complexion. Deep-set eyes and full lips complemented her rich Eastern European accent, transfixing me as she began her litany of new patient questions.

"So what brings you to see me today? Oh, I see you're a referral from your sister. You have the same eyes."

"I need to get something for mood," I started, hoping we wouldn't have to go too far down the psychotherapy path with my whole life story of feeling like a sinking ship. "I've been on Zoloft for a long time but stopped seeing the psychiatrist who prescribed it because the medicine made me feel too numb all the time. And the visits were too expensive and I felt I was starting to repeat myself and didn't need to talk about stuff any longer." I could feel my voice starting to break and my eyes welled up against my will.

Her gaze didn't leave my face as she listened intently.

"I thought I could manage okay without the medication so I didn't take it anymore—haven't had it for almost six months now. But I've got a really stressful job and I'm having a difficult time keeping my composure at the office." By now the tears were streaming down my face, my words sticking in my throat. "I just don't know what else to do anymore. I feel so hopeless and, at the same time, I know I have to get up every day and get to work."

"You need to be on the medication. It's the only thing that will keep you from feeling so sad. But there are new drugs, cleaner drugs with less troubling side effects than the Zoloft."

She started me on Lexapro, one of those kinder, gentler drugs she predicted would soothe my troubled spirit. After two months I went back to her feeling no worse, but certainly no better. We checked Lexapro off the list of possibilities.

She then wrote me a prescription for PaxilCR, assuring me the side effects of this drug wouldn't be as numbing as Zoloft, and said, "You should feel better in no time." She was right. Within a few days I felt pretty darn happy. My leaky eyes subsided and my energy level increased—still a bit numb around the edges, but clearly in a better place than I'd experienced for quite some time. The pills were pink and my mood matched them.

By this time the Internet began its takeover of the advertising industry. Everyone's job required inescapable aspects of the bits and bytes of producing marketing magic in confounding ways. I bravely jumped on that digital bandwagon when a man I worked with during the snail mail days offered me a position at his newly launched dot-com agency. The challenge of forging a new career in a world wrenching itself from the confines of ink-on-paper fueled my ambitions. I loved the new technologies, and sitting alongside the new young marketing wizards in client meetings made me feel as if I had a whole new world at my fingertips. Unfortunately, the stress levels imposed by the inherent learning curve sapped my brain of neurotransmitters and put me on an emotional tightrope.

Over the course of the next five years, to combat the pressure and inherent nagging depressive feelings, I maxed out the milligram dosage of the PaxilCR, which started at 12.5 mg and ended up at 50 mg. I persisted with complaints a few months later about needing a stronger dosage.

"Doctor, I still don't feel right. I'm always on the verge of crying and I think I need you to up the Paxil a little more."

She shook her head and sighed heavily. "I can't give you any more. Why don't you stay with your current dosage and try meditating." Her once sympathetic understanding of my condition suddenly felt diminished. I don't know who felt more frustrated with my lack of progress, but I silently scoffed at the idea of meditation. Whenever I tried meditating, I kept falling asleep because I felt so depressed, and sleep was a handy alternative to being sadly awake. It seemed ironic that one simple letter constituted the difference between the two therapies. Swap out the "c" in medication for the "t" in meditation and maybe I would feel better. I left her office without a new prescription, convinced I'd figure out a way to soldier on.

Dr. T suggested I keep a bottle of Xanax handy for times of increased distress. She included a warning that I should take a Xanax only in extreme instances of anxiety, as this was a "dangerous drug."

"You can become dependent on this medication, and withdrawal can be a big problem," she dutifully informed me. I took her advice seriously and only availed myself of Xanax on one or two occasions, just as a test drive. But consciously I felt afraid of becoming addicted to anything so powerful as to be categorized "dangerous." My vigilant caution unwittingly set up my life's exit strategy when I squirreled away the twenty-eight remaining tablets and unconsciously planned for "a rainy day."

Over the next few years and unbeknownst to me, Paxil, the medication I relied on to prop me up, lost its efficacy even as I religiously swallowed the tiny pink pill every morning. I ultimately assumed all the unhappiness I felt was "just me"—a miserable, ungrateful wretch of a woman. How dare I feel so sad when I've got everything going for me—health, family, a great job. *Jeeeezus, Martha, what the hell else do you need in life?*

I soon decided the nightly pours of vodka, Scotch, or chardonnay could fill in where the Paxil fell short—the Frick and Frack of my own self-prescribed solution. There was simply no way to escape the need to escape.

~∽

My bottle of Paxil didn't make it to the emergency room the night of my overdose of Xanax. I subsequently went cold turkey with no antidepressant while I lay in an emotional pit in Saint Vincent's medical unit. Not until a week later in Reiss 2, my third day on the psychiatric ward, did anyone offer me a psychotropic hall pass—EffexorXR. When Dr. G's intern officiously handed me several pages detailing dosage, side effects, and the usual precautions while taking Effexor, I responded with gloomy resignation, knowing I'd be back on another monthly schedule of doctor visits to get the little slip of prescription paper—my ticket to ride on the medication merry-go-round. I got the ride part, but the merry definitely eluded me.

My stand-in psychiatrist at Silver Hill continued the Effexor initiated by Saint Vincent's, plus an added hit of Lamictal as a mood stabilizer, even though my mood couldn't have been more stable—as in low, down, and flat. I didn't ask any questions about an official diagnosis, or which drug did what; nor did anyone bother to explain each pill's secret ingredient. I simply sucked them down every morning when the nurse pinched them into my outstretched hand with the accompanying Dixie cup of water while I patiently waited for the magic to begin, presumably within two weeks.

Post-discharge from Silver Hill, six weeks came and went with no lift from the drugs, no easement of pain, but a noticeable increasing hopelessness managed to burrow its way into my heart. The up side of feeling so down and out was this: I lacked the vision to expect anything good happening, so Effexor's failure to bring me to a happy place didn't disappoint me. I figured the ongoing sadness defined the status quo. I lost all expectations for a normal life and resigned myself to living with an undercurrent of gloom.

∾

The early spring months following my hospital stay kept me busy with doctor appointments, therapy sessions, and watching the clock to make sure I didn't forget to take my pills at the correct time. After the first month I noticed the Effexor the hospital prescribed was nearly gone.

When I asked my psychotherapist at the Life Awareness Center to write me a refill prescription, he told me I needed a psychiatrist to do that.

In my gross naiveté I asked, "You mean you guys can't do that here?"

"No, we just handle the talk therapy here. And the drug rehab meetings. You'll need to find your own psychiatrist for your meds."

"Oh, great—so now I've got to schedule another appointment on my depression dance card," I replied. Keeping up with all the meetings and medication times looked like a full-time job that I felt too exhausted to tackle. I wondered if and where it would ever end.

I had no choice but to go back to my notes from Silver Hill and call the psychiatrist in Connecticut they had recommended. I had stubbornly clung to hopes of returning to work in the city where a New York doctor would be more convenient. My job loss and subsequent decision to leave New York made Dr. S my obvious recourse.

Our first appointment got off on a weird footing when he insisted I drop my connection with all providers in New York. This included a talk therapist I'd seen several times on recommendation from Silver Hill after my release. I'd been making progress with Francine and I didn't want to abandon our blossoming patient/therapist relationship. I felt caught off balance and slightly intimidated by Dr. S's seemingly unfair demand.

"I have to know everything about your medications in conjunction with your psychotherapy. You need to see one of our therapists in this practice so we can confer on a weekly basis."

He spoke with an authority bolstered by an exotic accent from somewhere on the other side of the world. My intuition growled from somewhere way down in my gut, but I knew I needed him as the doctor to write a monthly script for the much-needed medications, so I acquiesced.

He wore a dark, expensive, three-piece suit and his shoes were shinier than a Marine sergeant's. Everything about his office pointed to efficient, up-to-date, and competent. The furniture even smelled new. His modern desk was built with shiny chrome and thick spotless glass. The only problem with it was that it didn't face me. The doctor, his chair, and his desk faced the door, perpendicular to where I sat on a small love seat against the wall. Consequently, he never even had to look at me. He sat across the room, deftly entering notes on an electronic tablet with a stylus while I offered up my story for the umpteenth time.

I feebly rationalized my lingering reservations about severing my other therapy ties. *Maybe he's the guy who might be really "taking charge" of my care and wants full ownership of my mental health.* I knew I desperately needed an anchor, someone who would steer the ship and get me out of the rough, uncharted waters I felt roiling around me.

He tactfully wrapped up our session with, "Here, Mrs. Rhodes. Take these samples, and here's a prescription for you to fill. Follow these instructions and I'll see you in two weeks. Just be sure to follow the directions I've given you very carefully. These drugs are powerful and you need to introduce them gradually to your system or you'll run the risk of seizures."

I walked out of that first visit with Dr. S armed with a fistful of prescriptions for Concerta, stronger EffexorXR, and increased dosage instructions for Lamictal. The complicated instruction card he scribbled out for the three drugs required discipline and focus. The responsibility overwhelmed me.

I took great pains to follow the instructions to the letter, cutting pills in half and marking the calendar religiously to follow the rules of gradual progressive dosage. Over the following three months, an entire section of the kitchen counter became the staging area for my army of bottles filled with drugs ascribed to the treatment of illnesses ranging from attention deficit disorder, bipolar and unipolar depression, schizophrenia, manic depression, obsessive compulsive disorder, post traumatic stress disorder, and epilepsy, to name a few. After a couple of months we ditched the EffexorXR and gave Topamax and Seroquel a shot at pulling me out of the emotional sludge. He threw in a bottle of Klonopin with hopes of quelling my increasing anxiety about not feeling any relief. Then we opted to try Abilify as a helper pill to boost the original antidepressant pill that was supposed to help but didn't.

My twice-monthly appointments boiled down to what felt like a game of "Pin the Tail on the Depression Donkey." The thirty- to forty-five-minute wait for an appointment—to which I always arrived on time—only added to my anxiety. Chronic double-booking of patients by the appointment scheduler and miscommunications or non-communication by the administrative assistants infuriated me. The less-than-ten-minute consultations with Dr. S gave me the opportunity to state—in a one-way conversation with him—how miserable I felt. After he jotted down everything I said on his computerized writing tablet, barely looking up at me, he concluded our brief encounters by handing me another armful of pharmaceutical samples and scrawled sheets from his script pad. He didn't seem to have an answer to my question, "Doctor, what's my diagnosis? What's wrong with me?" although the wide variety of medications and combinations of the drugs he prescribed left me thinking that I was nothing more than a woebegone work-in-progress—a "To Be Determined" at best.

Titrating up and down with the various medications created an emotional and physical roller coaster ride for me, particularly with the move from Effexor to Seroquel. Unfortunately for me, and for those around me, one of the side effects of coming off Effexor is increased agitation. It was so powerful that the Martha we all knew morphed into a person whose personality and behavior became disturbingly unrecognizable and at times downright frightening.

In fact, a normally pleasant ferry ride across Long Island Sound from Connecticut that July Fourth weekend brought the drama of the threatening side effects to center stage.

Our son had invited us to a baseball tournament where his teams were slated to compete. Since John and I both love the game at all levels—youth, college, semi-professional, and the major leagues—we decided to treat ourselves to a weekend getaway from the tedium of my illness. Although depression robbed me of focus, and medications failed to sharpen that tool, I took it upon myself to put this little travel project together for us by planning the route, the hotel, and everything in between. I felt invigorated to have an assignment where my project planning skills would once again be useful for something—anything.

Information for hotels, restaurants, and even Fourth of July fireworks displays on Long Island were easy to find on the Internet. I compared hotel reviews, checked out maps for proximity to the ball fields, and printed out a list of appealing eateries. The biggest challenge would be the holiday traffic on the infamous Long Island Expressway. In a moment of sheer brilliance, I came up with the idea of taking the ferry from Bridgeport, Connecticut, across the water to Port Jefferson, Long Island.

I thought to myself, "We won't have to sit in traffic," and (I began to wax poetic here) "we can enjoy the sun on our skin and the wind in our hair."

I logged onto the Bridgeport Ferry website to make a last-minute car reservation for the busy holiday weekend. Carefully reviewing the driving directions to the dock, departure schedule, and pre-boarding requirements, I booked a round-trip ticket for us, feeling quite smug that I added this nautical amusement to our weekend adventure.

Our Saturday morning departure went smoothly—I had us packed up with MapQuest directions printed out, overnight bags, a healthy breakfast for the ferry ride, and a hearty picnic lunch for the ball game. My attention to detail and ability to stay on schedule impressed me beyond even my own expectations.

We arrived in Bridgeport in plenty of time to be the first car in line as we jockeyed our way onto the automobile boarding ramp. I kept the manila travel folder holding all the travel maps and reservation information within handy reach as the crew member directed our car into the bowels of the vessel.

Shortly after we pulled away from the dock, a loud, garbled voice on the public address speaker blared out, "All drivers must leave their vehicles and to go to the upper deck to obtain their tickets."

Since I'd paid by credit card when I made the reservation online, I shrugged to John and, with my travel-planner mind set, I assured him, "Don't worry, honey, I've got the reservation receipt. I'll go upstairs and sort it out."

After standing on a long line observing how the tedious ticketing procedure operated, I approached the window fully confident that I had everything in order—automobile reservation confirmation, payment receipt, and passenger IDs. The crisp nautical uniforms worn by the two men taking fares and handing out tickets belied their lack of professional demeanor.

"How many passengers in your car?" one of the men curtly asked me without looking up from his register.

I blinked at his question, confused and a little put off by his brusqueness. I immediately opened my trusty file folder loaded with evidence that I didn't need to buy a ticket.

"Excuse me, but I made the reservation online and here's my receipt. Do you need to see the credit card I used?"

"I asked you a question, ma'am—how many passengers in your car?" His impatience began to compete with my sense of being organized and, well, in the right.

"There are two of us, but that shouldn't matter—I've already paid for the car and here's the receipt."

Again, he ignored my carefully produced documentation, which only frustrated me further since his uncooperative, officious attitude gave me no hint as to what the problem could possibly be. I ungraciously made up my mind that he was wrong about everything and I, of course, was completely in the right.

"You need to purchase tickets for passengers."

"Do you mean to tell me the charge for the car carrying the passengers who drove that car onto this boat doesn't include their fare? I didn't see anything about this when I made the reservation on the website. "

"Well, it's ON the website, lady, and you have to pay for passenger tickets."

Perhaps my mental state skewed my perceptions, but I could have sworn he sneered at me. He suddenly became a short, bald, rude bully who, with his shitty attitude, set a match to my short fuse. I felt my face flush and the hair on my scalp tingled. In that moment, all my careful planning, all my dotted "i's" and crossed "t's" went up in smoke before my eyes.

"I read your website very carefully. I went over every bit of the schedule and the different boats and the instructions about showing up thirty minutes before boarding time and what to do if I had to cancel and, and, and…"

By this time he gave me such attitude my slow-burning fuse reached the explosive and I went after this guy with a verbal barrage of what an asshole he was and he was in the wrong job if he thought taking care of customers meant treating them like idiots and he could just go fuck himself.

"And by the way, it's NOT on your fucking website, you fucking moron."

I slammed the twenty-four bucks into the little pass-through hole and snatched up the tickets he shoved back at me. If not for the Plexiglas barrier between us, I might very well have climbed over the counter and grabbed his scruffy throat.

Shaking and completely stunned by my own hideous behavior, I descended the stairs and found my way through the dark hold of the ferry and back to the car. The upbeat, adventurous woman who had left him only fifteen minutes earlier now fell into John's arms weeping, screaming, sobbing.

"I thought I had done everything perfectly, I can't believe I missed that detail about passengers in cars needing additional tickets, and how could I have been so stupid and how could I let this upset me so much and what a mess I've suddenly made of our holiday trip."

He sat with me, speechless and equally shaken by the storm created within his happy-wife-turned-maniac. His usual response to all of my meltdowns was silence—partly because he knew from experience the storm would pass and trying to do anything would be like throwing gasoline on a bonfire. But I also think my intense reaction to things frightened him. He didn't know what to do with me or for me, so his best plan of action was to simply do nothing.

It wouldn't have surprised anyone who witnessed the exchange upstairs at the ticket office if a paddy wagon awaited us on the New York side of the crossing. By the time we rolled our car off the ship, my hysteria had drained me so thoroughly I couldn't show my face in public. I felt so disgusted with myself that feigning social pleasantries was all the more loathsome.

"Please, just take me to the hotel. I can't go to the ball field. You'll have to explain to Nicholas that I'm not feeling well," I murmured to John. His sad eyes told me how disappointed he felt, not for himself and not for our getaway weekend plans gone awry. His sadness rooted itself in realizing how helpless he was to do anything for me.

He didn't say a word until we finally got settled in our hotel room, where I curled up on the bed, exhausted and numb.

"Honey, please, I want to stay with you. I can't leave you like this."

"Why would you want to be with me when I can hardly stand being with myself?" I wept, turned my back to him and burrowed myself further into the pillows in a tight fetal position.

My shame and humiliation were so mortifying that I begged him to leave me alone. I felt too miserable to be with anyone, not even the man I loved more than he could ever know.

"Please, I just wish I could die. If I'd been struck with incurable cancer, everyone would understand and feel sorry for me and you'd all have to let me go, so why can't you all just let me die from this miserable depression?"

At that moment, my pain felt equal to—if not even more than—what I imagined any physical illness could pose. The constant anxiety, sadness, fear, and despair strangled me. I felt inexorably alone and as if I were dying a slow death of emotional asphyxiation. I may not have been diagnosed with incurable cancer of a vital organ, but I knew I was in the throes of battle with what felt like cancer of my soul.

I spent the rest of the day holed up in the hotel room— exhausted, ashamed, humiliated, angry, frustrated, and, above all, utterly without hope that I could go on living like this.

John went to the ball field without me. When he returned we stood in stilted silence at the full-length window of our tenth-floor hotel room watching distant fireworks illuminate the coasts of Long Island and Connecticut. The world outside celebrated life, liberty, and the pursuit of happiness as I secretly contemplated how I could escape my pernicious pain.

The following morning I cancelled the return tickets on the ferry and we drove the traffic-jammed length of the expressway back to Connecticut. I felt like a complete failure, wondering what was happening to me, and how and why John stayed married to me.

∿

For the rest of that summer guilt and a sense of responsibility compelled me to show my family that I'd give my best try to do my part in healing myself so that I could get on track, get another job, basically get myself back in the game of life. I made every effort to avoid the unwashed, unkempt, hangdog look that many depressed people exhibit. At the very least, I felt obligated to appear to be getting better, even though deep in my heart I knew the opposite to be true. Proof of that lay in the fact that every morning when my eyes opened (or even before they opened), an intense, inextinguishable wave of putrid dread would compete with the heavy blanket of hopelessness enveloping me, making it impossible to even lift my sluggish head from the pillow. I equated it to what I called "emotional nausea."

It's difficult to say if the side effect of the drug-of-the-moment caused me to sleep for sixteen hours out of the twenty-four, or if my own sloth and inability to muster the impetus to get myself out of the bed immobilized me. On the other hand, the side effects of the next prescription, Seraquel, left me wide-awake and unable to even nap for almost sixty hours over the course of one weekend. This same drug also sent me into more dramatic melt-downs of ranting and rage where, should I have found myself in a public place during one of these scary episodes, any on-duty cop would have been within perfect rights to haul me into the local lock-up. Fortunately, I had the presence of mind to warn John not to allow me to even go to the grocery store alone for fear I might explode like a weapon of mass destruction.

Soon after the infamous ferry ride, another unfortunate occurrence landed me in our neighborhood hospital emergency room with a fractured big toe—the result of a swift kick to a very heavy box that got in the way of my ranting one day. Three hours of waiting room time and about $1,800 later, I managed to hobble around for the next several weeks wearing one shoe, self-consciously accepting sympathy for my incapacitation, but secretly knowing I only had myself to blame for this regrettable circumstance.

As it turned out, this became my personal bottom-of-the-barrel moment. The next day, my throbbing big toe and I came to the indisputable conclusion that, not only were the drugs not helping me, they were altering my basic personality. For their tiny size and shape, manufactured in soothing pinks, yellows, and blues, I marveled at what a potent, negative change they inflicted on me. Every time I opened my mouth to deposit the seemingly innocuous little pellet, an eerie voice inside my head sounded a distinct warning: "Caution! Swallow at your own risk!"

At our next appointment, I summoned up the nerve to confront Dr. S, telling him that instead of feeling better since I became his patient, I felt worse—worse than I did the night I overdosed.

When I asked him, "With all these different drugs I've been taking, why don't I feel better? Why aren't they working after all this time? When am I ever going to be happy again?" his dismissive response left me dumbfounded.

"We have to try different drugs. This is an art, not a science!"

I left his office wondering why I had wasted almost six months as his living experiment, trusting him and his ability to lead me out of the dark cave that had become my life. I couldn't tell which feeling was stronger—disillusionment or undiluted rage.

As soon as I got home I went to the kitchen counter and, with one sweep of my arm, I dumped the entire array of prescription bottles into a brown paper bag. The drug-fest was over. So was the pity party. I immediately scheduled another appointment with Dr. S where I informed him I would no longer be taking any more antidepressants that he or anyone else prescribed. To his protestation, "You can't do that!" my response was immediate and uncensored.

"Doctor, during my last visit you told me this is an art, not a science. Now you need to know two things. One, I am not your canvas and, two, you are no Rembrandt."

I left his office proud and relieved that I had told him the truth, but completely unsure as to what my next steps would be. I felt lost with nowhere to go, no options for therapy that would get me back to a longed-for normal life.

∾

When I first went to Dr. S and he asked me to give up my New York psychotherapist, Francine, I felt disappointed—no, subliminally pissed off—to have to start all over again with a new person, rehashing all the drama with yet another professional who would nod, take notes, ponder, and with a crisp "Time's up" let me walk out the door with no answers. I didn't want to get off on the wrong foot with Dr. S, so I agreed to the switch, but in my heart I resented him for it.

I felt comfortable and validated with Francine. She had a contemporary, artsy, wise-woman way about her and I sensed she really listened to me, always asking me to tell her more. Her cool website showed me she ran a really "with it" practice. I hated to tell her my new doctor didn't endorse my seeing her in New York and him in Connecticut. During our last meeting she graciously and professionally conceded that she understood, but the unspoken message exchanged with our eyes told us otherwise.

My first visit with the new therapist, Susan, did not go very well. I'm sure she heaved one huge sigh of relief when my Evil Twin left her office that afternoon. I treated her with a crappier attitude than she deserved as I flaunted the proverbial "bug up my ass" and made no apologies for it. I made sure she knew I'd been foisted on her—or her on me, I'm not sure which—by Dr. S and that I resented having to give up Francine because of him. Nevertheless, we both knew we were stuck with each other.

By the end of our third appointment, I got over my indignation and surrendered to Susan's kindness, gentle support, intelligence, compassion, and, above all, open-mindedness. I began to rely on her for her keen insights, honest feedback, and, as needed, an occasional pat on the back for any minor successes I managed to achieve. She provided me with valuable scientific information about the cause and effects of major depressive disorder in addition to entrusting me with several books from her personal library.

Susan tactfully listened to my ever-increasing complaints about the inadequate care I experienced with my psychiatrist, whose pervasive ego took precedence over my needs as his patient. While he continued doling out medication trials, she treated me with genuine concern and expressed empathy for my growing list of worries about weight gain despite loss of appetite, agitation and anxiety, sleep deprivation, forgetfulness/memory loss, inability to focus, dull headaches, constipation, flatulence, clumsiness, and chronic muscle/back pain.

When I finally decided to go online and check out some of the drugs I'd been given, I discovered just how many of their side effects I had actually experienced. It would have been nice if drying up tears could have been one of them.

On the surface, my decision to stop taking all medications might be regarded as irrational, equal to the opposite—and extreme—action of overdosing on Xanax, but I saw myself on a maddening merry-go-round with no bright and stately horses on which to ride. If my body could not tolerate the burdensome side effects of taking the drugs, drugs that hardly put a dent in my depressive symptoms, I meant to find out what my body could tolerate without them.

In retrospect, I see the enormous risk I took and would not recommend it to anyone. Sudden and total cessation of antidepressants, as is the case with many other medicines, can lead to catastrophic reverberations such as seizures. At the time, however, a persistent survival instinct trumped my confidence that antidepressants would do me any good. I had given up on psychiatrist appointments and the ten-minute medicine meets. Mistrust, negativity, and unbounded frustration clouded any consideration to look for another doctor who might be a better caregiver. Other than continuing appointments with my talk therapist, Susan, I had essentially stranded myself on an island when I cut myself off from the traditional, well-traveled road of available drug treatment options.

Self-doubt versus gut instincts niggled at me as I sat at home wondering if I'd painted myself into a corner. As a result of my "just say no" decision, a tugging feeling of emotionality and tearfulness remained embedded in the back of my throat and in the top of my chest. This constant urge to cry resulted in dull headaches that created an irritable, testy disposition. I noticed that my memory or "mindfulness" increasingly waned.

I even forgot my sister's phone number, a number I had dialed countless times over twenty-five years. As I held the phone in my hand to call her, struggling as my fretful finger hovered over the keypad, fear sent me into a relentless crying jag. I anguished about the prospect of being stuck forever in this Godforsaken hopeless state. I had lost my edge and I missed it. My confidence in my ability to get things done, an attribute I always prided myself on, lay in serious jeopardy.

A desperate, sinking feeling warred with the strength I needed to fight it—like running in a dream or being trapped in quicksand. It felt like nervousness, fearfulness, hopelessness, agitation, and sorrow all pureed together, topped off with a sprinkling of paranoia.

Abandoning antidepressant medication reminded me of a bad breakup with a lover gone sour. Can't live with him—and cannot live without him. Damn him!

7 | CALL 1-800-TRY-TMS

Full-page ad in Connecticut Magazine:

August 2009

TREATING DEPRESSION WITH MAGNETIC STIMULATION

Physicians are Using the Newest Technology to
Treat Depression Without Discomfort or Drugs

My therapist, Susan, proved her commitment to my health care in gold the day I showed up with the magazine advertisement for Transcranial Magnetic Stimulation and she didn't shake her head. With an expression neither excited nor skeptical, she took the page from me and studied the ad's brief description.

"We are now offering the first Transcranial Magnetic Stimulation (TMS) in Connecticut. TMS, only recently approved by the FDA, is a new concept in fighting depression. As the patient sits comfortably in a chair, a painless electromagnetic current (similar to MRI) is applied to the scalp. This outpatient procedure has few side effects or risks, and is effective for depression. Put yourself in the most experienced hands. Choose a Hartford Hospital doctor. It could be the most important decision of your life."

"Hmmm, this sounds interesting. I haven't heard much about it, although I know it's been researched in patient trials. Are you thinking of trying TMS?"

"Yes, I've already called Hartford Hospital about it, actually. I know it's new and it sounds a little scary, but what've I got to lose? The FDA approved it, so that must mean something."

"Well, it can't hurt to have the conversation about it, especially since you haven't had any improvement with the meds."

Her open mindedness delighted me. For the first time in months I felt hopeful about the future.

"I'm kind of excited. I have an appointment next week with the doctor who's the head of the TMS center up there."

"Great! I'm anxious to hear what you find out. And I'm glad you're at least looking at options."

∽

By now, Susan and everyone close to me knew I had given up on the antidepressants several weeks earlier, and all were concerned as to how I should proceed. I had fired my first psychiatrist, who handed me off to another doctor in the same practice, Dr. R. He was younger and his initial approach to my illness seemed kinder and gentler. During our first appointment he listened to my frustration about medications with a knowing look and quiet nod. He seemed more open than Dr. S, but he was nonetheless committed to dispensing more medications in addition to some high-intensity vitamins. I wanted to develop a working relationship with this new doctor whom I hoped would help me, so I reluctantly acquiesced to try more drugs, Abilify and Deplin, a high-intensity vitamin.

Other available major depressive disorder treatment options at that time were next to none. The only one I had heard of was Electroconvulsive Therapy (ECT), which, by its very name, gave me the shivers. I immediately discounted it due to its bad reputation for considerable memory loss, not to mention hideous depictions in Hollywood films such as *One Flew Over the Cuckoo's Nest*. It seemed barbaric and much too extreme to even consider. I've since found out that ECT has been dramatically improved, although the procedure still involves anesthesia and delivers an electric shock to the entire brain. Memory loss continues to be one of the side effects.

It was during the two weeks while I waited for relief from the Abilify and Deplin that I discovered TMS. How I found out about it was nothing short of a miracle.

My sister had been flipping through *Connecticut Magazine* while awaiting a dental appointment when she serendipitously spotted the ad. She called me as soon as she got home.

"Hey, Martha, it's Maria. I found something that might help you with your depression. It's called TMS. I don't know anything about it, but the ad says it treats depression without drugs. It's FDA approved, too."

Borrowing one of our mom's old adages I quipped, "Any port in a storm. Would you fax it over so I can take a look?"

As soon as we hung up the phone, the ad came through on my home office fax machine. I suddenly felt as if I had discovered a hidden clue in a mystery novel and the key to the plot was waiting for me on the next page.

At my next psychiatric appointment I planned to ask Dr. R if he thought I should try TMS since by that time it was clear the Abilify and Deplin weren't helping me.

"Doctor R, I just found out about a new treatment called Transcranial Magnetic Stimulation. Do you know about it?"

"Well, yes, I do research at Columbia University and about ten years ago I participated in studies done on TMS…" he replied without going any further. His hesitation unnerved me. I couldn't tell if that was good news or not, so I pressed him.

"What do you think about it? Do you think I should try it?"

He immediately shook his head and cleared his throat as if to prepare me for a professorial mandate. "The studies haven't really proved TMS works any better than ECT, so I wouldn't recommend it at this time."

"I'd be afraid to try ECT anyway because of the memory loss factor," I said. "But I did some research on TMS and I'm interested in it since it's a therapy that doesn't involve medications or their side effects."

I put my purse on my lap and pulled out a file folder. "Here, I brought you a copy of a study I found online."

I handed him a nine-page printout of a clinical trial done in 2001 at the University of Illinois at Chicago's Department of Psychiatry.

I persisted.

"The study compared TMS versus ECT and TMS produced comparable therapeutic results in severely depressed patients."

He leaned back in his chair and crossed his arms over his chest without taking the folder that I held suspended in mid-air. "No, no, I'm familiar with all the TMS studies. I don't recommend it and I don't think you need ECT either."

"Then, if the medications aren't working and you don't think TMS or ECT are options for me, what am I supposed to do?"

"Just stay with the antidepressants and eventually, hopefully, we'll find something that will help you." He looked at his watch as he shifted his weight in his chair, expecting I'd get the message that our time was up.

I got the hint. Our time was more than "up". I left his office without making my next appointment. I intended to pursue TMS regardless of what Dr. R thought of it past, present, or future. He couldn't offer me hope or even a hint of medical advice to assuage my depression. He was taking me down the same path of trial-and-error medication therapy as the other doctors.

I got in my car and left the parking lot, simmering with indignation. *Why shouldn't I find out about TMS on my own? It's been seven months since I crashed and burned and there's no relief in sight. What the hell do I have to lose at this point?*

As soon as I got home I placed the first call to Hartford Hospital's Institute of Living.

A friendly voice answered, "Hartford Hospital Institute of Living. May I help you?"

"Yes, I'm looking for information about Transcranial Magnetic Stimulation."

"Sure, I can help you. Of course, you'll want to set up an appointment with our TMS director, Dr. K, but before you do that, I need to ask you a few preliminary questions."

She launched into a litany of queries about metal objects.

"Do you have any metal in your head and do you have any implanted devices such as an ear implant, a pacemaker, defibrillator, or insulin pump?"

Suddenly I got the impression there might be a hitch to qualifying for the treatment. I happily responded "No" to all questions, but then screeched to a halt with, "No, wait, I do have metal in my head—I almost forgot, I have a tooth implant. Will that make me ineligible?"

"No, tooth implants are fine because they're made with titanium. It's only ferrous metals we have to worry about because of the magnets."

I listened attentively, answering as calmly and accurately as I could, but to have stumbled upon a therapy for depression that didn't involve drugs had me jumping out of my skin with excitement. Before we completed the phone call, the interviewer also informed me I would have to drive more than an hour to Hartford five days a week for four to six weeks. I was ready to travel to the moon.

∽

In a weird way, not taking any drugs felt like a vacation from a tedious job. I no longer had to worry about what time I took the first one and at what dosage, and then remember what time I had to take the next one, or wrack my brain to remember if, in fact, I had actually taken the damn thing that morning. At first I found myself going to the kitchen counter, once covered with pill bottles, only to stop and remember that I had relieved myself of this daily task. This freedom felt similar to when I quit smoking cigarettes some forty years earlier. I'd keep reaching for the pack and have to remind myself, "Oh, I don't do that anymore—how terrific." Nevertheless, without any medicine, I felt trapped by darkness, fretfulness, and despair.

Within a week I was sitting in Dr. K's spacious and comfortable office at Hartford Hospital's Institute of Living. It felt more like a living room than a doctor's office. Tastefully upholstered chairs rested on a thick carpet. An attractive table lamp warmed the room with a gentle ambient light instead of the usual institutional overhead fluorescents. Rather than peering at me from behind her large mahogany desk, Dr. K took a seat close to me where we could see each other's faces without distraction.

At first I couldn't take my eyes off her. Her short auburn hairdo framed her dark eyes. She was outfitted in a perfectly tailored tweed suit that looked as if it came from a couture designer and not a local department store. She spoke with a deep voice that made her natural beauty even more striking.

I perched myself on the edge of the leather couch, although its comfortable cushions begged me to sit back and relax. With my elbows dug into my knees, both palms supporting my tired head, my mind raced as I tried to get a sense of whether this could be my new life line, not wanting to miss a single word this calm, soft-spoken doctor was about to share with me. My nervousness and fear of the unknown competed with blind hope that a practically unheard-of therapy could be the real solution for my severe depression.

"So why have you come to find out about TMS?"

She opened the floodgates for my account of years of depression, stressful jobs, a challenging family life past and present, my suicide attempt with subsequent hospitalization, and the ultimate failure of drug treatments.

Dr. K listened with an attentiveness that instantly disarmed me. I couldn't hold back my tears. Since my disastrous escapade with Xanax, I had not received so much time and empathy from any other psychiatrist. We spent more than an hour discussing my history and how TMS could help me.

"Is it like Electroconvulsive Therapy? Because if it is, I don't think I can do that—it seems too scary and I heard it can cause memory loss."

"No, TMS doesn't involve electricity or shocking your brain like ECT. It delivers magnetic pulses on your outer scalp, right here," as she held her hand to the left side of her head. "The pulses activate electrical impulses inside your brain, but it's very gentle and noninvasive."

Any anxiety or doubts I walked in with about trying an alternative therapy began to vaporize along with my tears. The doctor explained in digestible, yet technically appropriate terms, how the procedure is performed in an office where the patient sits comfortably in a chair while an electromagnetic current is applied to the scalp, similar to an MRI but with no claustrophobic environment. The MRI-strength magnetic pulses stimulate nerve cells in the areas of the brain that regulate mood, specifically the left prefrontal cortex. These activated cells then communicate with the pathways to the area of the brain that releases neurotransmitters. The release of these neurotransmitters helps to decrease symptoms of depression.

The simplicity and logic enthralled me. Kind of like the vegetable juice commercial where the actor smacks himself alongside his head and exclaims, "I coulda had a V-8!"

Dr. K continued explaining. "The pulsed magnetic current is painless, although I will admit, initially, some patients experience tenderness on the scalp site where the magnetic pulse is applied. But don't let that worry you. I have patients who take a couple of ibuprofen prior to treatment to alleviate any discomfort. And most patients become accustomed to the sensation in just a few visits."

"If I have to come every day from so far away, how long does each session last?" Already I started planning logistics.

"You'll come for your first session, which will take about an hour and a half so we can set up your program. But after that, you'll be in and out of here in less than forty-five minutes."

She paused a moment and then looked me straight in the eye when she said, "The success of TMS, however, depends on the patient's commitment to showing up five days a week for four to six weeks."

I heard her caution loud and clear. Since the hospital is more than an hour from my home, I weighed the reality of traveling back and forth in a car for over three hours every day for six straight weeks to sit in a chair for forty-five minutes.

"Would I be able to drive myself or would I need someone to take me?" I asked.

She answered unequivocally, "You can drive yourself back and forth from every treatment—unless you just want someone to keep you company in the car."

"Will I have to worry about side effects after every treatment?"

"No, you won't have any side effects at all. In fact, some patients experience an increase in energy after their treatment," she assured me.

Dr. K pointedly warned me that TMS is not a quick fix for depression. She indicated that many patients don't see improvement in their depression symptoms until two to three weeks into the treatment regime. I did the math—that's ten to fifteen sessions, I figured. As I sat there listening, my heart sank just a little and I wondered if this would be yet another wasted block of precious time spent foolishly pursuing the Holy Grail of Depression Cures.

She leaned forward in her chair and with an empathetic, confident, and reassuring manner, she quickly dispelled any doubt in my mind when she added, "After about fifteen visits you should start to feel better. Some of my patients say they get a feeling of lightness. Others describe it as a heavy weight being lifted off their shoulders or as if the cloud of depression just vanished."

Dr. K's description captured my imagination. I felt like a child at story time as I listened intently while she described other patients' experiences with TMS. I envisioned a dark, heavy rain cloud hovering over my head, following me as if I were bound by a long, invisible leash, unable to detach from it no matter in which direction I moved. Suddenly a light wind passed under it, severed the cord, and carried the dark cloud far up into the sky.

Her final question stirred me out of my fantasy and back to our conversation.

"I think you would be an excellent candidate for TMS. What do you think about doing it?"

"I honestly think I'm ready to try it. Nothing else seems to be helping, and after my horrible experience in the hospital, I never want to end up there again."

A sense of relief overwhelmed me. I knew in my heart I was in exactly the right place. Here was a real doctor in a real hospital, offering me a real solution to my very real symptoms of debilitating depression. She successfully convinced me that, although it was a new technology, TMS was approved by the U.S. Food and Drug Administration, and it was safe, noninvasive, and painless. I appreciated the fact that I wasn't being sucked into a sales pitch, and her expressed confidence in TMS and its more than fifty percent success rate only increased my resolve to learn more about it when I got home to my computer.

Not until I reached for my purse and started to leave did I remember to ask two very important questions.

"How much does this treatment cost?"

"Depending on how many sessions you need, it costs between $8,000 and $12,000. You should plan on the higher amount, though."

I paused before asking the deal-breaker question.

"And does insurance cover it?"

She lowered her eyes and shook her head. "No, not at this time, unfortunately. The insurance companies still want to call it experimental. They'll pay for ECT, but not TMS. But we can submit paperwork for you and try to get it approved. Sometimes they'll reimburse the patient after the treatment."

I was so intent on finding help for my depression that the idea it would cost too much—or at the very least not even be covered by insurance—immediately braced the four sides of square one, the box I'd hoped to be out of by the end of this appointment. I thanked Dr. K for her time and left her office.

As I handed over my co-payment check, the administrative assistant at the front desk offered me a blank insurance request form to fill out before I left the office.

"Just fill in the information on this application and we'll submit it to your insurance company right away," she said.

I spent several minutes placing check marks next to my personal information, medical conditions, and medications history. When I handed it back to her through the glass window I asked, "How long does it usually take to get pre-approval?"

She took the completed pages from me and avoided my anxious eyes. I couldn't tell whether her quick, abrupt movement and brief response meant she was really busy or maybe was just her way of quelling my premature hopes for insurance coverage.

"About three weeks. They'll send you a letter and copy us here in the office."

It sounded like she was reciting a "routine procedure" script, which hinted to me that this was not a slam-dunk case of an insurance company giving the nod to $12,000 worth of treatments. I left the appointment, however, with a naiveté swathed in unabashed optimism.

Our health insurance policy had always covered everything we needed over the years. We frequently applauded our good fortune to have the comprehensive and generous benefits plan that John's job offered. Even though our family historically enjoyed excellent health, whenever any of us got sick, the insurance always came through. It didn't seem possible that now, when I needed it most, I wouldn't have coverage.

Unemployed, with no viable job options on the horizon and in the throes of surviving a serious depressive episode, taking on a financial burden so huge seemed like a very bad idea. And what if we spent all that money and TMS didn't work, just like the medications didn't?

I headed for home, wondering if I should stop at the corner bodega and pick up a lottery ticket. Suddenly, everything looked like a gamble to me—TMS, insurance, and my life.

8 | INSURANCE CHALLENGES

"Start by doing what's necessary; then do what's possible; and suddenly you are doing the impossible."

– Francis of Assisi

About a month after Dr. K's office submitted the request for coverage, the first denial arrived from my insurance company as a standard, impersonal form letter stating "TMS Therapy is considered experimental and investigational and is not medically necessary for your condition."

In retrospect I've wondered if the terms "experimental and investigational" were intentionally designed to instill hesitancy, fear, and doubt in the hearts and minds of the easily thwarted. Even for myself, I had to stop and consider the word "experimental."

You know, it's your frickin' brain, Martha—what if they zap it and something goes wrong? What if this TMS thing is still experimental and investigational enough that you end up a zombie because the magnets went haywire?

But then I realized I felt like a zombie already, so it really didn't matter. The denial letter only compelled me to dig deeper, to read everything available about TMS: how it worked, success or failure statistics, where it was being offered, and what kind of patients were getting it.

Several months later I discovered from an insurance liaison and patient advocate that, for the most part, insurance companies rely on ninety percent of people who have been denied coverage to just give up and go away. Providers are prepared to spend the money for the other ten percent of folks who challenge their decisions and who have the mental—no, emotional—fortitude to persevere through the appeal process. It's a basic numbers game.

As early as when I was seeing Dr. R, and even before I went to Hartford and received my first denial from the insurance company, I had begun my research into TMS—my conscious stab at positive thinking. I found a 2001 study done by the Department of Psychiatry, University of Illinois–Chicago School of Medicine that concluded, "A 2-4 week randomized prospective trial comparing [repetitive] TMS to ECT produced comparable therapeutic effects in severely depressed patients."

TMS had absolutely no side effects compared to those of ECT—with short-term memory loss being the most onerous one. The no-side-effects part was a huge "bingo" for me. If I could receive a treatment that relieved the pain of depression without so much as an ounce of gained weight and with no nausea, sleeplessness, irritability, or gastrointestinal disturbance, I wanted it. What could have been construed as throwing caution to the wind was, on the contrary, wind in my sail of finding a way out of my misery.

Although crestfallen by the first denial letter, I remained convinced TMS was worth pursuing, since by then I had been off all antidepressants for almost three months and precariously balanced myself on a tightrope strung between two poles of hopefulness and complete despair.

On a scale of one to ten, my energy level lingered at about a three. I usually slumbered in the arms of Morpheus anywhere from twelve to sixteen hours per day. My only impetus to get out of bed centered around my shame at John returning from work only to find me in the same place he'd left me earlier that morning.

If I did manage to get out of bed before noon, I cried almost every morning, all the while yearning for night to settle in so I could escape into my dreams, which by this time had become my sole source of entertainment. All social activities, outside interests, even phone calls were automatically dismissed. I continued to keep weekly appointments with my psychotherapist, whose unfailing support of my pursuit of TMS fueled the notion that I could actually fight the insurance company's position and get them to reverse the decision.

At that time, Neuronetics was the only company with an FDA approved TMS system called NeuroStar TMS Therapy®. Neuronetics provided patients with a third-party patient/insurance liaison service called NeuroStar Care Connections (NCC). A patient representative guided patients through the insurance appeal process with help writing letters, supplying research data, and overall keeping the patient's paperwork in order to avoid missing the strict deadlines imposed by the insurance companies. They worked with the prescribing doctors and their patients to make the TMS experience, and subsequent expense reimbursement, as seamless as possible. (Since that time, however, the prescribing doctors are handling this within their practices.)

When my NeuroStar Care Connections representative called to tell me my appeal could take three to four months, I wanted to collapse. I expected six weeks, maybe a couple of months, but not that long. In my mind, every day felt like climbing a mountain. My usually dependable game face wore thin, and at times my resolve to live seemed as fleeting as a cloud on a windy day. With zero options, unless I wanted to surrender to ECT, I steadied myself with, "Just proceed, Martha. Just proceed."

NeuroStar Care Connection emailed me their response letter draft shortly after the insurance company's first denial, about eight weeks after my initial TMS consultation with Dr. K. It detailed all the scientific information about TMS, citing various studies that had been done, remission rates, and the overall symptoms of treatment-resistant depression. It was a good start and represented me fairly and accurately, but I sensed something was still missing.

The Care Connection letter didn't convey what I, the patient, really felt and how my life was on a downward spiral because of my illness. Instinctively, I knew the insurance people who were reviewing my case would need to understand more about me as a person before they would grant me coverage. I decided then and there I would be the only one who could effectively convince them to reverse their denial.

Thus began my indefatigable letter-writing campaign to make my case for insurance coverage for TMS.

My strategy was three-fold, all based upon insurance companies' willingness to pay for Electroconvulsive Therapy and not TMS. First, I wanted to present the scientific facts about TMS and its proven success, especially since it received FDA approval. Second, I planned to supply financial implications of TMS versus ECT, plus the perpetual expense of doctors' appointments and medications. And finally, I would plead the case for my own medical need with the written support of my doctors and therapist.

I carefully edited the businesslike, scientific tone of the Care Connection letters into a more reader-friendly version. I rearranged the information, making sure that the very last paragraph conveyed in my own voice what living in my skin was really like—day in and day out, hour-by-hour and minute-to-minute. I emphasized how difficult my untreated depression was for my family and how that dynamic furthered my decline.

No one could have been more surprised than I to discover I could actually sit down at a computer and organize my thoughts as clearly as I did. I developed an unquenchable thirst for verifiable data and anecdotal information. I began this quest in October and continued my evidentiary dig for another six months. During that time I received a second denial letter bearing the exact same verbiage as the first, at which point I launched an even stronger investigative case questioning why insurance should automatically cover Electroconvulsive Therapy and not cover Transcranial Magnetic Stimulation.

It also occurred to me how patently illogical the reasoning behind their denial seemed in light of evidence to the contrary. In response to the evaluation done by Blue Cross Blue Shield deeming TMS therapy to be an inefficacious treatment, I gathered supporting research on the Internet, citing TMS safety and its success rates with patients suffering from major depressive disorder. Unfortunately, there wasn't much information available to the general public, but I unearthed professional peer-reviewed literature that gave me a well-balanced assessment of the technology. My main agenda focused on safety, efficacy, durability, and sustainability of remission from depression.

NeuroStar TMS Therapy System® received FDA clearance in October 2008. The approval was based on trials completed for adult patients suffering from major depressive disorder who failed to achieve satisfactory improvement from one prior antidepressant medication of adequate dose and duration. The clinical study included patients with non-psychotic, unipolar major depressive disorder (MDD) who had suffered previous depressive episodes and had extensive medication treatment histories without satisfactory improvement. At this point, I had already tried (and failed) with five different antidepressants, and my mood stayed at normal or below, which eliminated me from the bipolar camp. I wasn't psychotic and I was historically depressed, so I passed muster on all counts.

FDA approval of this product was a lengthy and rigorous process to ensure its safety and effectiveness. I applauded the FDA's responsibility for protecting and advancing public health and assuring the safety, usefulness, and security of products it reviews. But I persisted in requesting an explanation as to why an FDA-approved treatment, specifically designed for depression, could still be considered "not medically necessary" by my insurance plan in light of the FDA's blessing.

I mentioned this in my appeal letters particularly since the safety and efficacy for ECT treatment was on a very close par with TMS. I couldn't find any research indicating that ECT was otherwise more effective and/or safer than TMS. Nor did I find any research that supported the premise that ECT was a preferred therapy over TMS.

ECT is more invasive, requires general anesthesia with its inherent risks, and has cognitive side effects including memory loss. TMS is performed in an outpatient setting that does not require anesthesia and hence allows patients to return to their home or work immediately after treatment.

Unlike ECT, TMS does not compromise a patient's short- or long-term memory. TMS has none of the side effects many patients experience with medications, such as weight gain or sexual dysfunction.

The only serious side effect mentioned in the literature for TMS is an insignificant chance for seizure. Surprisingly, antidepressants can induce seizures at an even greater risk than TMS. According to a study published in the *Journal of Clinical Psychiatry* in 2008, the estimated risk of seizure under ordinary TMS therapy is approximately 1 in 30,000 treatments (0.003 percent of treatments), which is 1 in 1,000 based on a TMS six-week treatment course. (0.1 percent of patients). The risk of seizure for patients taking prescribed medications can range from .1 percent to up to 2.6 percent.

Most important, studies have proved that TMS has a comparable success rate to ECT in non-psychotic patient trials, and the outcome for TMS patients is as predictable (or unpredictable, for that matter) as ECT.

The only difference I could surmise from the insurance company's point of view was that ECT had been around longer. Could that be the only reason ECT therapy merited coverage? If so, then I offered the notion that not all patients who are unresponsive to medication need the degree of invasive therapy that ECT imposes.

My sense of caution, however, was not subverted by a

desire for a positive outcome with just any treatment. Perhaps the inference of "experimental procedure" in the denial letters somehow haunted me. Nevertheless, I remained prudently optimistic while delving into the details of the technology, spending much time researching the pros and cons of TMS, and discovering extensive clinical literature supporting its use for patients with major depressive disorder.

Before gaining FDA approval, the manufacturer conducted six-week duration clinical studies. More than 10,000 active treatments were safely performed on patients with treatment-resistant major depressive disorder. The following results were observed:

- The primary efficacy measure, the Montgomery-Asberg Depression Rating Scale (MADRS), symptom score change at four weeks was statistically significant compared to a placebo. Similar results were observed with the Hamilton Depression Rating Scale (HAM-D).
- Treated patients had statistically significant response and remission rates, which were approximately twice the rate of placebo-treated patients.
- TMS therapy also produced statistically significant improvements compared to a placebo on the HAM-D factor scores for core depression symptoms, anxiety symptoms, somatization, and psychomotor retardation.
- The treatments were safe with no systemic side effects such as weight gain, sexual dysfunction, nausea, or dry mouth.
- No adverse effects on concentration or memory were present.
- No seizures occurred.
- There were no TMS device versus drug interactions.
- Some scalp pain or discomfort during the therapy occurred but declined markedly after the first week of treatment.
- Less than five percent discontinuation rate occurred due to adverse events from TMS treatment.

Since FDA approval, TMS is now being offered to treat

depression successfully at approximately 400 clinical locations across the country, including major institutions such as the Mayo Clinic, Columbia, Duke, and Harvard Universities, and Walter Reed Army Hospital. As to success rates, in a yearlong study performed by the manufacturer, patients being treated with the Neurostar TMS system throughout the U.S. have shown a response rate of 58 percent, and a remission rate of 37 percent. Over 250,000 treatments have been administered as of this printing.

In a press release in February 2009, Lt. Col. Geoffrey Grammer, MD, Chief of Inpatient Psychiatry at Walter Reed, stated that twenty-four patients had been treated with TMS at Walter Reed so far, and that five hundred TMS procedures had safely taken place. Most patients showed an excellent response to the treatment and experienced relief from their depressive symptoms. Dr. Grammer acknowledged that TMS had practically no side effects, no risk of long-term health concerns, and high efficacy ratings. He stated that TMS could potentially extinguish the remaining barriers that inhibit service members from seeking mental health treatment.

"Having TMS demonstrates the Military's willingness to bring cutting-edge technology and care to the best patients in the world, our Warriors," Dr. Grammer said. "Most importantly, we now have a new option to treat patients who have not responded to medications that has minimal side effects and a large margin of safety."

Although I had initial, albeit temporary, positive results with Zoloft and PaxilCR, they eventually ceased to alleviate my depression symptoms. My subsequent therapy attempts with Seroquel, Abilify, Lamictal, Concerta, Lexapro, and EffexorXR gave me no significant relief. In some cases, the side effects were too steep a price to pay, even if I had received some benefit. I always followed the recommended dosages for adequate periods of time but continued to have symptoms of anxiety, hopelessness, suicidal ideation, lack of interest, and overall inertia. I knew I could not continue my life without pursuing treatment for my depression, but I definitely knew I had given antidepressant medications more than a fair chance to help me over the many years of suffering.

Because of my treatment history, my psychotherapist and doctor agreed with my decision to seek TMS therapy, because it had been proven to be effective in cases such as mine. I could not accept how an insurance company's decision should outweigh those of medically trained and clinically experienced doctors who actually knew me, and who could see how threatening depression was to my life.

I also failed to understand how a more expensive treatment known to cause cognitive deficits was covered by insurance, while a less expensive, noninvasive, non-anesthetic treatment like TMS was not. Supporting the second prong of my challenge strategy, I pointed out how the cost of both ECT and TMS were comparable. In fact, per treatment session, ECT is more expensive than TMS due to the costs incurred with the anesthesiologist. My insurance company had already paid $24,000 for hospitalization, medications, and psychiatric treatment at the time I began my challenge for coverage. This didn't include the medical and pharmacy claims related to my depression prior to this particular episode. Going forward I could not imagine what the costs would be, but the sum of past, present, and future claims would certainly outweigh the cost of TMS.

In addition to the efficacy and financial viewpoints, I needed to impress upon the approval board that I was at a dead end with treatment for depression. I explained that I had always considered myself to be a person of courage and fortitude. My career as a successful professional proved this. These attributes steadily declined over the years as my depression increased with my brain's inability to produce the necessary chemicals to support my mental health.

I described how I found myself living in a world where there was no escape from the daily worry of self-harm and constant sadness. I lived in a world where I had to manufacture a false smile when I could easily burst into tears. I pretended to be happy so I wouldn't worry my family and friends who knew of my depression and who felt helpless to do anything about it. I lived in a world where I felt constant guilt that I simply didn't have the faculties to embrace their love and support because my brain refused to operate in a way that made it possible. I lived in a world of fear—fear that the hopelessness and darkness would win out. Fear that I would lose my ability to endure life with this debilitating condition.

Categorizing TMS as experimental, investigational, and therefore not medically necessary was unfair to someone who had tried with no success to be helped with medications that even the doctors admitted to being experimental in their own practices of psychiatry. My doctor's claims that finding a successful medication for me was "an art, not a science" reinforced this. Couldn't this approach be considered experimental as well? If so, then why not cover "experimental and investigational" TMS?

The medical and mental health professionals have admitted that comparatively little is known about the human brain and mental illness. This seemed to me to be all the more reason why alternative treatment should be supported and included in the pursuit of successful mental health care.

The more I researched and wrote, the more determined I became to get TMS treatment. Family and friends were respectful enough to limit their inquiries about my progress in the fight. This helped to alleviate the pressure I had already placed on myself to win the battle. Outwardly, I maintained an attitude of expecting a victorious outcome. Inwardly, I worried incessantly that I would become a loser in the insurance company's own lopsided game— The Numbers Game.

9 | Lost in the Stars

You do not have to sit outside in the dark. If, however, you want
to look at the stars, you will find that darkness is necessary.
But the stars neither require nor demand it.

> – Annie Dillard, *Teaching a Stone to Talk*

Dogs should pee before they go to sleep at night. At least that's what my copy of *Doggies for Dummies* told me. Which is why I found myself standing under a dark mantle of summer sky around nine o'clock every evening with our newly adopted shelter dog, Josie.

In the beginning, neither of us knew what to do with each other. I wasn't raised with animals—seven kids crammed into a two-bedroom house curbed any fleeting desire for a family pet my mother might have allowed—so I didn't know how to even walk a dog properly. Josie's sketchy beginnings in her neglectful first home followed by several months in the limbo of a rescue shelter left her just as confused about her current life as I was about my own.

Some days I thought I was feeling a little better, but by the time I went outside at night with Josie, I always shrank under the vastness of the mysterious darkness of outer space. Its enormity minimized any sense that I mattered, either to myself or to the world around me. The insignificance I felt in the face of the cosmos smothered my spirit whenever I gazed up at the billions of stars. I tortured myself with a litany of futile questions. *What's out there? Is there another pitiful soul on some other planet looking out and asking the same questions I'm asking, like, is there a God? And if there is*

128

a God, why did he put me here, and if there is someone else out there, what does it matter to either of us anyway?

I never felt more hopeless than during those few minutes tending to a little dog's bladder business.

Josie's mixed breed of Terrier and Chihuahua outfitted her with eighteen pounds of irresistible cuteness. Her soulful brown eyes set against her champagne-colored coat stole our hearts the moment John and I met her at the Save-A-Dog shelter. She had been up for adoption for several months, and although the staff warned us of her behavior issues, her adorable appearance outweighed any possibility we would not take her home with us.

Ostensibly, her assigned mission was to keep me company and distract me from my woes. Looking back on the situation, I think getting me out of bed in the morning ultimately became her more important job. Josie became my new alarm clock, and there was no snooze button when her persistent barking roused me to tend to her morning constitution. I'd drag myself out of bed, prepare her food, and then take her for a stroll down the little lane behind our house.

Our morning walk often required more energy than I thought I could manufacture. She was there to keep me alive, while I still wished I could die. More than once while we traipsed along the busier main road, I secretly wished a car racing past us would just hit me from behind and end it all. But then I stopped my morbid ideation with the worry that I might not have enough time to let go of the leash so Josie could run away and not get hurt. Realizing how much I actually cared for her put a damper on my morose fantasy. The "Let's Save Martha with a Puppy" plan began to work.

The report from the animal shelter indicated Josie had spent most of her first eighteen months confined to a crate, and according to the shelter staff and our veterinarian, she also demonstrated signs of physical abuse. Her temperament flared with palpable mistrust of anyone on either two or four legs. A couple of outings at a local dog park where she snarled at—and attempted to bite—other dogs and their owners proved to us that the warnings about Josie's issues were indeed real.

On one of our early trips to the dog park, I immediately discovered how dog people naturally want to be friends with other dogs and their owners. Total strangers greeted me with a pleasant "Hello" and a welcoming nod. Josie, on the other hand, displayed aggression and antisocial behavior to dogs and humans alike the moment I closed the interior gate. Her back hairs shot up and she maintained a low volume growl whenever another dog came near for a sociable sniff.

Two Birkenstock-clad women chatted me up with genuine interest about Josie.

"Oh, he's so cute—how old is he?"

"Uh, her name's Josie and he's a she. Two years old, I think, but I'm not sure."

They looked at each other quizzically. I quickly added, "We got her from a shelter. They couldn't give us a definite birth date."

"Oh, how wonderful she came from a shelter. Good for you. There are so many abandoned dogs who need a good home."

I appreciated the hero effect that being a dog rescuer automatically bestowed upon me, although it was pretty obvious to everyone I didn't know what I was doing or how to handle Josie, especially when she responded to their admiration with her pointy little teeth and accompanying growl and I recoiled in nervous anxiety. I secretly commiserated with Josie, since we both shared the same unpredictable volatility.

"You know, you can take her to the local Family Y for dog training," one of the women offered. The other lady gave me a card for a certified dog behaviorist. I stuck it in my pocket wondering how much money this little dog was going to set us back—on top of my own psychotherapy bills.

A tall, wiry gentleman introduced his Dachshund, Joey, and a very large Doberman named Princess. I've always been afraid of big dogs, probably because a large, black mongrel jumped in my face when I was a toddler and scared the living dog chow out of me. Besides, Dobermans have dubious, albeit unfair, reputations from the way they've been portrayed in the media. But Princess dispelled my worries. She was calm, elegant, and obedient to her master. Above all, she didn't show any aggression or misplaced interest in any of the other dogs. I surprised myself by petting her with guarded enthusiasm.

Overhearing my conversation with the other women, the Doberman's daddy stepped in to make friends with Josie with unabashed self-confidence. I figured if he could handle a big dog like Princess, who by now sat adoringly at my feet, then he probably knew the trick to dealing with my psycho dog.

"Be careful," I warned. "She's a nipper and you can't reach down to her."

Of course, as soon as he went to pet cute little Josie, she jumped up and bit him faster than a desert rattlesnake. "I'm so sorry, I, I … are you bleeding?" I didn't want to hear his answer.

Obviously he was. He pulled a clean white hanky from his back pocket, wrapped it around his forefinger, and gently escorted his mild-mannered Princess off to another part of the yard. I packed Josie into the car and cried all the way home. I knew I wouldn't be going back to that dog park, or any other public place for that matter. I didn't know how to deal with her unpredictable behavior and, in any event, I didn't want to get sued for it.

My deepest sadness, however, was the pity I felt for Josie. Dog parks are supposed to be fun. Normal dogs love playing outside with each other. She's going to be alone all by herself because she can't be around people or other dogs. What fun will that be for a cute little dog? I felt genuinely sorry for her.

Not too much further down the road it occurred to me I might be feeling sorry for myself as well.

The upside of Josie's antisocial behavior meant we couldn't really invite anyone—friends or family, and certainly not strangers—to our house. When John suggested we hold off on hosting a summer barbecue with friends, I jumped to an immediate "Yes!" and sighed with relief. This fit in neatly with my own antisocial leanings, so in that regard, Josie and I were a perfect match.

I longed to have her be a well-balanced normal dog. But my inexperience with pets revealed how sorely I lacked the skills to rehabilitate a dog afflicted with what our dog professional diagnosed as acute fear aggression. When some dogs are fearful, they retreat from threatening situations by hiding in a corner or under a table. Others respond to their fear by lashing out with barking, nipping, and in some cases attacking. But both sides of the behavior coin are based in a visceral, instinctual fear.

I felt sick when I thought about her abusive past. I felt even sorrier that she now lived in such a neurotic, anxious state of mind. I wished I could somehow erase all the anxiety her life's circumstances imprinted on her little doggie brain, where she felt she had to fight for her life even though she now lived in a completely safe and loving home.

I soon realized that Josie and I were dog-paddling in the same dark waters. Sink or swim. *Who's helping whom here?* After three months of hauling myself out of bed to tend to her morning needs, my patience wore thin trying to deal with her unpredictable episodes of freaking out over benign things like a passing bicyclist or a UPS truck, and predictably nipping at anyone who reached to give her a loving touch. Several times she turned on John and me with a yelp and a nip if we happened to unwittingly startle her.

My sympathy for her nervous condition was at odds with my impatience with it. I thought to myself (with only a twinge of guilt), *Now I know why they got rid of her. Now I know why she spent so many months in that shelter.* Eventually, her shortcomings became my shortcomings. I began to look at her lack of progress as another personal failure.

After two months of religiously watching *The Dog Whisperer* on cable television, subscribing to several dog-training website newsletters, and attending a dog behavior seminar, I seriously doubted we could keep her. As intensely difficult as our adjustment proved to be, however, the idea of taking Josie back to the shelter signified much more to me than a failure to communicate with an eighteen-pound pooch. Her breakdown and mine became inextricably connected. Her unsuccessful adjustment to a loving, attentive family paralleled my own seeming lack of a benevolent fate. I uncontrollably sniped at my loving husband, whose patience rivaled biblical Job's. I shut out my own circle of love and support by ignoring family and friends. I didn't return phone calls from them, nor did I ever reach out to ask for their help when I felt so low and hopeless.

So every night before ending the day, Josie and I stood there under the stars as a pair of peas in the same pitiful pod—both of us sniffing out what our next move should be, wondering how we ended up on the end of the leash—whether we liked it or not.

Two things kept me on track with this little creature. Number one—Josie made me laugh as only a winsome pup could. The second—despite my crankiness, short temper, and severe lack of decorum with the rest of the world caused by the depression—she periodically reminded me that a well-meaning, nice person, one who could lovingly care for a helpless little dog in need of a good home, still lived deep down inside me. Clearly, Josie provided me with a dose of antidepressant that didn't come from the local pharmacy.

∽

As the weeks crawled by waiting for word about TMS insurance coverage, Susan, my ever wise and compassionate therapist, expressed delight when I told her we added Josie to my cache of survival tactics.

"What a great idea—and walking the dog every day will get you out of the house and exercising."

"Josie's a really cute dog, but she's loaded with behavior issues.

She's got fear aggression and I'm not sure I'm emotionally equipped to handle them."

Susan could see I was floundering, and since I'd stopped all medication, her concern for me increased. She paused a beat before she asked me pointedly, "Martha, what are you going to do if a final denial from your insurance company arrives in the mail? What's your Plan B?"

I appreciated her concern, but the fact that her optimism seemed to be waning didn't bode well for my goal in getting TMS treatment. I thought for a minute and realized my optimism never allowed me to consider anything but a successful outcome.

"I don't have a Plan B. I don't know what I'll do."

"Why don't you take another look at trying ECT?" She reached over to her desk and handed me a magazine. "Here's an article I saved for you from Sunday's paper. It's Carrie Fisher's experience with ECT. She described how it saved her life and how she's suffered with depression for years."

Susan's suggestion of taking a second look at ECT fell on my deaf ears, and Princess Leia's endorsement didn't sway me. A few weeks earlier I dared myself to watch a public television documentary on mental illness that depicted an actual ECT treatment. It horrified me to the point of tears. The voice-over described how the patient was told she would feel better in eight or nine visits. The documentary followed her through an entire summer of trips to a hospital where she surrendered her anesthetized brain to twice as many induced seizures as her doctors had anticipated with no apparent success or hope for relief.

The procedure itself seemed extreme, despite the reporter's claims that great strides have been made to minimize the treatment's invasiveness. I wasn't buying it. The memory-loss side effect was the deal-breaker for me. After her ECT session, the girl seemed flat and listless. She also found it difficult to recall what had happened to her the previous day. If I wanted to have memory lapses, I'd just as soon go back to drinking myself into a vodka stupor. ECT therapy also meant returning to a hospital and depending on someone to drive me back and forth for treatments—none of which suited my independent nature.

I opted to remain a player in the waiting game. My final insurance appeal letter lay in the hands of an external third-party review panel—unbiased and separate from the insurance company adjudicators. Fortunately for me, Connecticut's insurance laws required this step in the appeal process once a patient received a second denial. I took the tack of detached confidence, putting it all in the "hands of God," although by this time my depression had obscured any belief in even the concept of a god.

The late summer moved into autumn and then winter while I lingered in my personal holding pattern. Optimism and fatalism constantly sparred with one another. When I'd take Josie outside to the yard each night for her final pee-patrol, looking up at the expanse of inky sky so distinctly punctuated with countless stars, I continued to imagine how my significance on earth paled in comparison to the vastness of the heavens. I frequently found myself humming the title song from Kurt Weill's Broadway musical, *Lost in the Stars*, whose story is based on hope, despair, and a crisis of faith. The sentiment in the lyrics about how we humans are so randomly lost in the universe—out among the stars as if we are blowing around in the darkness—resonated in my mind as a nightly anthem.

I reminisced how, as a little girl, my dad took me outside one starry summer night to teach me about the Big and Little Dippers. He bent down and put his face next to mine so our eyes looked out together. He extended his long arm and pointed up to the vast sky.

"Look for the brightest stars, Martha, and you'll see three stars that form a curved handle, and then follow the curve down to see four more stars that make up the bowl. Do you see them?"

"Yes! I see the curve—I see the handle! Oh, and now I see the bowl, too!"

"That's the Big Dipper. Now look at the two outside stars on the bowl and follow with your eyes just a little ways out and then up. They point to the curved handle of the Little Dipper. And the star at the very end of the Little Dipper's handle is called the North Star, the most important star in the sky. All the other stars move around, but the North Star always stays in the same place. You can count on it."

It was magical being out under the stars with my father, whom I adored. Having him show me that the sky held some abstract, yet visible meaning made me feel special, as if he was sharing a heavenly mystery with only me. There are big secrets in the sky, I marveled, mesmerized by how smart my dad was to know about them.

Years later when I got to high school I learned that the Big Dipper played an important role in the abolitionist movement during the Civil War. The Big Dipper's bowl pointing to the North Star's steadfast position helped slaves navigate their escape to Canada. The folk tune "Follow the Drinking Gourd" became a code song within the Underground Railroad because the Big Dipper resembled one. The lyrics reminded runaway slaves to follow the drinking gourd and they'd find freedom.

Fifty years after my father showed it to me, I stood beneath those same stars. My eyes trained on the bowl, I followed the two pointer stars to the Little Dipper's handle. I closed my eyes and prayed to the North Star. *Please, please help me find freedom from the pain I'm in.*

I was counting on it.

10 | Unhappy Holidays and a Trip to Paradise

"… My accident really taught me just one thing: the only way to go on is to go on. To say 'I can do this' even when you know you can't."

– Stephen King, Duma Key

As the days shortened, I braced myself for the holiday season, knowing my jubilant spirit lay as dormant as a hibernating black bear. It pained me to even think about the social demands I'd either have to force myself to rise for, or find a way to gracefully excuse myself.

John decided to move Thanksgiving dinner to our bachelor son Nicholas's place. For years it was a robust feast at our house with twelve or more people vying for elbowroom around our table—a spread overflowing with dishes of homemade everything. This year, we graciously declined offers from the same friends and relatives who had always been at our home. My dark mood would be an unwelcome guest at anyone's table. John and I managed to transport a small turkey with a few baked potatoes, some frozen corn, and a can of jellied cranberry sauce. The three of us sat stiffly at our first Thanksgiving in more than thirty years away from home, not knowing what to say or feel. I did my best to keep from crying at the dismal excuse of a turkey dinner, a perfect reflection of my state of mind.

The nostalgic Christmas music CDs I always pulled out the day after Thanksgiving remained in their plastic cases. *John Denver and the Muppets, The Cambridge Singers,* and *The Texas Boys' Choir's*

Favorite Carols would have to wait for another Yuletide when I could listen without feeling as if they were funeral dirges. Any Christmas gift shopping I managed to do for John and the kids happened on the Internet. My favorite holiday activity of wrapping gifts with colorful paper and a Christmas purist's red and green satin ribbons never happened. I felt either too exhausted or emotionally incapable to feign the merriness of that Christmas.

By New Year's Eve 2009 my modus operandi had nothing to do with living, yet everything to do with surviving. The winter months passed as I holed up in my house cave, mindlessly biding time while awaiting a final verdict from the insurance company. I had essentially resigned myself to living life as if I wasn't there— as if every flavor was vanilla, every color beige, every sound a muffled monotone voice repeating the same old tired advice, "Just keep going. Stay positive. Be hopeful."

By March I became impatient with waiting for a warm spring day and decided a visit with our daughter, Elizabeth, in Miami would assuage my lethargy. She'd called to let us know she had entered another triathlon and encouraged me to come down to cheer her on. I hoped the sun's rays would provide me with a natural mood lift, not to mention a little color in my pallid complexion.

I realized the last time Elizabeth and I had been together was the day she left me in the psych ward. Since Elizabeth's work schedule prevented her from coming home at Christmas, I felt even more separated from her. There was so much distance between us—physically and emotionally. I wondered if she'd had time to ponder what I'd done to myself with the overdose and if she now felt less forgiving. Her glowing face greeting me as I came down the airport escalator took away my worries.

I marveled at what a picture—masterpiece—of health and exquisite beauty my thirty-something daughter had become. She had tucked her mane of blonde waves neatly under her Miami Beach Ocean Rescue cap, which gave her a cute and sassy appearance.

Her broad athletic shoulders and deliciously tanned arms reached for my carry-on bag the moment I stepped off the escalator. She immediately launched into a welcoming string of chatter.

"*Hola*, Mommy! How was your flight? You're right on time. I've got a wonderful week planned for us. After the race on Sunday I'm taking a vacation day on Monday and I'm treating both of us to a spa day at the Standard Hotel. We're gonna get massages and have lunch and sit by the pool all afternoon."

Her energy amazed me. I envied her enthusiasm, her authentic lust for life.

"Sounds good, honey. I just hope I can keep up with you."

∽

During the first few days of my visit, I busied myself with reorganizing her kitchen, rearranging the cabinets with all the baking needs in one, all the canned goods in another. I fixed hearty, homemade meals, reminiscent of the mother who once prepared them with regularity—chicken cacciatore, tuna noodle casserole (her childhood favorite), and an aromatic apple crisp.

I discovered that it seemed much easier to build a "To Do" list down in Miami, away from the house I'd been neglecting in Connecticut for almost a year. I made a few trips to the local hardware store and home goods outlets for a variety of projects to keep myself occupied—a broken cabinet handle, sticking slider door, frayed rug edge. Fixing someone else's problems seemed more doable than mending my own 1,400 miles away.

Race Day arrived the following weekend. We woke up at 5:00 AM. Elizabeth's pre-race preparations fascinated me as she methodically mixed her energy drink, assembled her cycling and running gear, and made sure her participant number was properly displayed. She planned to do the Olympic version of the triathlon, a level above the beginner's Sprint category, but not the highest level, Professional. I felt nervous for her but refrained from any conversation other than to wish her good luck.

We got to the beach by dawn. I stood agog in the midst of at least two thousand people of all ages, genders, sizes, shapes, and fitness levels as the sun nudged itself over the ocean's distant edge. Loud music pumped adrenaline into the air as swimmers stretched their muscles, expelling any nervousness by flailing their arms and shaking their hands and feet. A Latina woman belted out the National Anthem from a raised platform, and a local radio personality thanked everyone for coming from all around the country to participate in the race. Daylight spread over the cool early morning sand and tension peaked as the opening ceremony culminated with the first blast of a bullhorn.

According to their gender and age, swimmers jumped into the water as human waves, one group after another, until the entire oceanfront percolated with white water, kicking feet, and arching arms pulling each racer along for the triathlon's first phase, a one-mile swim. I surrendered to the moment, forgetting all my troubles as I became instantly caught up in the excitement of watching such extraordinary effort. These athletes had trained for months for this one day. Most were competing with themselves; few even considered a place on the winners' podium after the one-mile swim, twenty-five-mile bike ride, and six-mile run. They were in it to simply do it. To be able to look in the mirror and know they had given their all to something as physically, emotionally, and mentally challenging as a triathlon. And there were thousands of them.

I ran up the beach and stood alongside the throngs of other spectators, all of us whooping and hollering for each athlete chasing his or her dream as they emerged from the water, pacing themselves as they trekked along the path to mount their bicycles for the second leg of the race. I noticed how they didn't respond to the crowd, how each athlete's discipline engraved a concentration in their eyes that tuned out everything except for what they had to do next to stay in the race.

I envied their ability to be so resolutely alone in the moment in spite of the crowd's cheers. Their focused faces expressed how they understood no one could finish this race for them. They had to do it on their own. I knew I'd probably never do one, but at that moment, I felt like I lived in a triathlon every day. I had plenty of cheerleaders of my own—my husband, my kids, my family and friends—but none of them could do my race for me. Although I was only a spectator that day, the athletes inspired me to find my own sense of purpose, find my pace, and get back in the race of my life.

∿

The day after the triathlon, Elizabeth kept her promise for the spa day at a trendy Miami Beach boutique hotel. We'd finished our massages by mid-morning and spent another heavenly hour languishing between the sauna and steam rooms. We then settled ourselves poolside, comfortably overlooking Biscayne Bay. I brought along a best-selling novel to dive into. The setting was idyllic, so devoid of stress and sadness, at that moment I felt as if life itself was fiction. The soft breeze and friendly sun endorsed my decision to escape reality—at least for that one day.

"This is just perfect, Elizabeth. Thank you so much for spoiling your old mom with this relaxing treat." I settled myself into a comfortable chaise lounge. Reluctantly, I removed my thick terrycloth spa robe. It felt like a soft cocoon, but I couldn't deny my body the sun's inviting gentle rays.

Elizabeth murmured something from a neighboring chaise lounge. "Mmmm … It's okay, Mom. You're very welcome." She had already reclined her overworked muscles from the previous day's race—where she landed a spot on the winners' podium—well on her way to a catnap. I took my cue and sat back to absorb the warm Florida sunshine. I adjusted the chair's back and opened my book, hoping to give my imagination something to chew on. Unfortunately, I couldn't concentrate enough to get past the first few pages, a symptom common to depression. I closed my eyes and pretended I lived in Miami all the time without a care in the world. Distant hushed voices from couples on the other side of the pool lulled me into a meditative state while a swimmer created a rhythmic splash, splash, splash as he cut through the crystalline water doing laps.

About an hour later a handsome young waiter arrived with our pre-ordered spa lunches. Just as he set the healthy salads in front of us, my cell phone broke the spell of poolside serenity. I instantly regretted having opted for the ringtone similar to the *Jeopardy* theme song. I fumbled for it in the depths of what felt like my bottomless bag, desperately hoping the loud ringing hadn't disturbed everyone around me. *Who the hell could be calling me here anyway? God this noise is embarrassing.* Just before voice mail could intercept the call I grabbed the phone and without looking at the caller ID, I hit the answer button.

"Hello?" I kept my voice low, still worrying about disrupting the peaceful atmosphere.

John's voice surprised me since he rarely called during the day. I assumed he wanted to see how things were going for the two favorite women in his life. My heart literally halted when he announced, "Honey, I just got home and picked up the mail. There's a letter here from the insurance company."

My ears buzzed and everything around me froze—the breeze toying with my book's opened pages, the couple splashing at each other in the pool, the sound of motorboats on the bay—as if someone hit the "pause" button on the DVD player. I couldn't speak.

"Do you want me to open it?" His hushed, somber tone revealed his concern for ruining my little vacation with bad news.

"Yes, please. I need to know now." I could hardly breathe as I sat straight up in the chaise lounge, straddling it like a horse going into the final battle.

My heart throbbed so loudly and my mind raced so fast, I didn't hear the first few words of the correspondence. I sensed dread and tension in John's voice as he began.

"This case was referred to an outside consultant, who is

Board Certified in Psychiatry. Following a complete review of the medical documentation provided, it was the reviewer's recommendation to overturn and approve the Transcranial Magnetic Therapy (TMS) treatment in this case. The reviewer's recommendation has been accepted and the denial of benefits has been overturned. The basis of this decision is that the additional information provided supports the medical necessity of the proposed treatment in this case."

As he read the rest of the letter, the word "overturned" gripped my gut. My face burned and every cell in my arms and legs vibrated. I choked back tears of joy, trying to avoid making an emotional scene in this placid, public place. Of course, to Elizabeth, my dramatic reaction only signaled something terrible had happened. She sat up abruptly and stared at me.

"Mom, are you okay? Did someone die? What happened?"

"No, honey, everything's fine. Everything's going to be fine. It's a good thing. I'm crying because I'm so happy."

On the other end of the phone John heard me reassuring her. He knew how much this meant to me, how much it meant to all of us.

"Congratulations, Martha. I'm so proud of you and how you fought for this treatment. You're courageous and I love you for it."

I didn't want to hang up the phone but I could tell that John felt he'd said all he could for the moment. I wanted to hear the words again. I wanted to make sure it was true.

"Call me later and read the letter to me again, okay?"

"Sure, honey. Let's talk about it after you get back from your spa day. Take care of Elizabeth now and I'll call you tonight."

As I explained to Elizabeth that I would finally be getting treatment for my depression with TMS, I almost didn't believe the words myself. I kept repeating over and over aloud, "I did it, I did it—I'm really going to have this therapy. The insurance is going to cover it and I'm really going to get better."

I don't think Elizabeth truly understood the magnitude of what was happening. She hadn't been around for all the endless months of letter writing, waiting, phone calls, and incessant worry. But watching me suddenly come back to life by a simple phone call must have given her hope that she'd have her mom back again.

After my conversation with John, and reassuring Elizabeth I was fine, I slipped into the swimming pool. With eyes closed and a smile on my relaxed face, I lay on my back, letting my arms and legs float languidly in the clear water. This must be how the athletes felt yesterday when they crossed the finish line. The bobbing motion kept rhythm as these words repeated over and over in my mind: I did it. I won. I did it. I won.

As soon as we got back to Elizabeth's place that afternoon, I called Hartford Hospital to set up my first TMS session. The nurse recommended I get a complete physical before starting treatments since I hadn't had one in over a year. The reason I hadn't had a physical seemed obvious. I didn't give a damn if my body needed curing for anything. In fact, I secretly hoped I'd get cancer and die, so bothering with a physical exam seemed counterproductive to that end.

"Shit, another delay," I thought to myself, but I hung up the phone and immediately contacted my long-time primary care physician's office in Connecticut.

I didn't recognize the receptionist's voice when she answered.

"Doctor's office, this is Melanie. May I help you?"

"Hi, this is Martha Rhodes and I need to get a complete physical next week."

"I'm sorry, Ms. Rhodes, but we can't get you in for six weeks."
She must be new—she doesn't know me like the regular receptionist does.

"Please speak with Dr. T and see if she can get me in sooner. It's important that I see her within the week. I need a procedure at Hartford Hospital that depends on it." *God, I've been her patient for so many years—surely she'll understand and give me a break.*

My insistence paid off. In less than a week after I returned from Miami, I sat in her office in a paper examination gown—

naked and shivering, but extremely happy. My urgent request, however, piqued my doctor's interest. As she fastened the blood pressure cuff around my arm, I effusively thanked her for fitting me in and yammered on about my pending TMS treatment.

She cocked her head, "And what's this TMS? I've never heard of it—educate me!"

Unable to hide my enthusiasm about having an alternative to taking the medications she had always so confidently doled out to me, I described it in as much detail as I could.

"It's a magnetic coil that delivers fast pulses to the left prefrontal cortex lobe of my brain. It'll stimulate the under-functioning pathways to increase the production of neurotransmitters." I hoped I was describing it accurately. Moreover, I hoped she wouldn't push back with some scientific data and burst my enthusiasm bubble. She listened with what seemed like professional interest as I extolled how noninvasive and safe TMS was, that it's a new, FDA-approved technology, and how I would be able to finally get some relief from depression without the drugs doctors had been prescribing for me for so many years.

Her surprising comment, delivered in her rich accent, left me almost speechless. "Well, it sounds pretty scary to me!"

Without missing a beat, I unabashedly proclaimed, "Doctor, I'll tell you what's scary—waking up every morning wishing I was dead—now that's scary!"

11 | First TMS Treatment

I shall be telling this with a sigh
Somewhere ages and ages hence:
Two roads diverged in a wood, and I—
I took the one less traveled by,
And that has made all the difference.

– Robert Frost, *The Road Not Taken*

Within a week I called Hartford Hospital to confirm they had received my health status report. Heart and blood pressure were A-okay. I was cleared to begin the treatments. I entered my start date for TMS on my calendar in bright red ink: "May 3, 2010" and underlined it with hopes for a brighter future. Several exclamation points completed the entry.

The drive on Interstate-84 to Hartford Hospital that Monday morning should have felt like a victory ride. After all, I had come so far with my decision to stop all medications and lived to tell the tale. I researched TMS in depth to make sure it wasn't high-tech snake oil. And I successfully campaigned for the money to pay for it in spite of a six-month purgatory of relentless depression symptoms. I had fought the good fight—internally and externally—and I had won.

Instead, as I prepared for the first TMS treatment session—vacillating over which outfit I should wear, packing the bulging document files I amassed during the six-month wait for this moment, fussing over makeup and hair—my emotions matched the gray, rainy day outside. Like salt in a wound, I felt as if I had a gloomy mood on top of the clinical depression. It might have been senseless anxiety over the logistics of actually getting there. Or perhaps a deeper, foreboding presence lurked with what felt like one of the biggest gambles of my life.

My trusted and devoted friend, Katherine, insisted on accompanying me on the inaugural trip. Katherine had known me for more than thirty years and was a stalwart supporter during some troublesome periods as I struggled to raise a family, maintain a healthy marriage, and pilot a challenging advertising career. Back in the early 1980s, Katherine spearheaded a support group we formed with five other women. She enthusiastically named us "The Rich and Famous Club." We met regularly to further our personal and professional goals, and we held each other accountable (sometimes painfully) on all levels.

Originally, we'd all set our sights on acting careers, although our separate journeys took three of us in other, nonetheless profitable directions. And even though Katherine emerged as a successful stage, television, and film actress, her extraordinary talents as a writer, director, and teacher continued to flourish. I always cherished her wisdom and insights, particularly her philosophy about "getting present" in one's body, something she taught to her acting students and also included in a self-help book she published.

Our history of mutual support is what made hiding my secret life of depression from her so much more difficult for either of us to understand. Even though I rushed to her for counsel on other traumatic events in my life (an acknowledgement of childhood molestation being one of the most devastating) I never shared the depths of my daily despair, nor did I reach out to Katherine during those murky death-wish moments. I have since come to learn that this charade is a common symptom of untreated severe depression and indicative of the dangerous level of hopelessness that accompanies it. Not until she heard the news of my suicide attempt did Katherine know the "real me," or rather, the really depressed me.

At first I resisted her offer to go with me for my first TMS session, as I had with my husband John's willingness to take a day off from work. My stoic attitude of "No, I'm really okay, I think I can do this myself, and I don't want to bother anyone", finally caved in to accepting her help. I figured my strict code of self-sufficiency hadn't served me so well over the past few years. It was time to admit that receiving another person's assistance might be a better strategy. Nevertheless, I insisted on doing the driving, unwilling to relinquish complete control. Katherine's positive attitude and unfailing friendship provided sufficient support from the passenger seat.

"So how are you feeling right now, Martha?"

"I don't know. Since I got the green light to do this, my mood took a nosedive, and I'm forgetting everything. Maybe because now that I know I'm getting the treatment, I've let my survival guard down. Maybe the good news of getting help came in the nick of time before I gave up on my life again."

During the hour-plus car ride, our conversation turned to talk of what I expected the TMS experience to be like, how it might feel, what the outcomes have been for others, and a myriad of fretful speculations. The closer we came to our destination, the stronger the F.U.D. factor pervaded my thoughts—Fear, Uncertainty, and Doubt—that the long-awaited messiah of relief just might not work. And then what would I do? For all the confidence I proclaimed to hold for this cutting-edge therapy, the sudden and unexpected attack of mistrust in its effectiveness gnawed at me. I wished I'd had the opportunity to speak to people who actually underwent the treatment—to ask them how it felt, if they were as scared to begin it as I felt now, and most important, did it work? The only information I had about TMS success came from the doctor I'd initially contacted and what little data I found on the Internet. Both maintained the response rate was approximately fifty percent, with thirty percent of patients achieving full remission from their depression symptoms.

I had no trepidation over whether it would hurt, or if I would feel weird side effects, or that since it was such a new procedure something could go drastically wrong. No, my biggest worry, the one that left me in a real sweat, was that I just might be one of the few patients that TMS failed to fix. By the time we pulled into the parking lot ninety minutes later, I had worked myself into a state of nervous, dubious anticipation. This must be what bungee jumpers feel like before they step off the 1,000 foot high bridge—nervous, excited, pumped up, and probably scared. But unlike bungee jumpers who do it for kicks, I was doing this for my life.

As Katherine and I entered the hospital building, a receptionist directed us to an elevator to take us to the second floor where the outpatient procedures took place. I noticed a few people drifting around in bedroom slippers and surmised this facility also housed live-in psychiatric patients. I shuddered as scenes from the Reiss 2 psych ward at Saint Vincent's flashed through my mind. I kept my eyes straight ahead and maintained my mechanical, even-paced walk toward the posted sign "ECT AND TMS THRU HERE"

We found the waiting room. It was small and empty, save for a flat-screen TV on the wall blasting the morning news. Just a few minutes passed before a sunny young woman emerged from around the corner, greeting me with a capable air that counterbalanced my increasing apprehension.

"Hi, are you Martha?" I nodded while she continued her introduction. "I'm Rosalind and I'll be your TMS coordinator. Come with me and we'll get you set up."

Unlike any other medical appointment I'd ever been to, I had no idea what to expect. I glanced at Katherine one last time as I left her to wait for me and turned to follow Rosalind like an obedient schoolgirl.

The atmosphere became dreamlike as Rosalind escorted me into a quiet room hosting a large chair similar to what you'd find in a high-tech dentist's office—or maybe a space ship, since a large computer with a long arm loomed over the back of it. A window filling the back wall needed help to light the room on such a dreary day. Fluorescent lights cast an austere ambience from the ceiling.

"Please put your earrings, necklace, rings, and watch in this little dish. I'll put them over here on the table where you can see them. You can't wear anything metal because the magnets in the TMS machine would detect them."

I climbed into the chair and wondered why I'd bothered to deck myself out with jewelry in the first place. A lingering habit to impress, I supposed.

Soon after, Dr. K, the psychiatrist with whom I'd met six months earlier, joined us. She explained in detail how she would determine the best, most effective place on my head to place the magnetic coil by performing a set-up procedure.

"We will be establishing what's called your 'motor threshold.' It will only take a few minutes," she assured me.

Rosalind placed two block-like foam cushions under my forearms resting on the chair's arms. "Are you comfortable in the chair or do you need to move back a little?"

I wiggled my lower back a little more snuggly in the chair and sat up a little straighter before I answered, "This is fine."

Dr. K continued explaining how she would establish my motor threshold by locating my brain's motor strip (the homunculus) that runs across the top of my head from left to right. From that, she would move the coil forward two to three centimeters and up and down on the left side of my head to find the spot in my left prefrontal cortex where the magnetic coil would ultimately be placed. After that, she would enter data into the computer and determine the degree of intensity and duration for the TMS treatments I would receive for the following six weeks.

As I listened attentively, my eyes welled up with tears, which took me completely by surprise. Rosalind reached for a box of Kleenex.

"I don't know why I'm crying," I blubbered through the

tissue, dabbing my eyes and nose. The doctor's and Rosalind's exchange of wordless, understanding expressions convinced me my reaction must have been expected and quite normal. Their compassionate nods and gentle reassurances invited my tears to flow even more freely.

"It's just that I've waited so long and come so far to finally sit in this chair and I hope it'll bring me back to normal."

I took a deep breath and felt my composure returning.

"I guess the anxiety and waiting for this day just hit me—but I'm so grateful to be here and I'm really sorry I'm such a mess right now."

Dr. K pressed my shoulder gently and spoke with quiet confidence. "It's okay, you'll feel better soon."

Rosalind handed me another tissue as she and the doctor adjusted the machine's arm hovering above my head.

I didn't know what to expect regarding the actual treatment, but thanks to Dr. K and Rosalind's confident demeanor, any doubt that I wouldn't be able to handle what originally felt like a calculated risk disappeared. I indulged myself with the idea that most people would not attempt this alternative treatment. Even though research had been ongoing for twenty years, TMS only received FDA approval eighteen months earlier. Most people would probably wait at least five years before trying something like this. I consoled myself by recalling the reaction I evoked from people when I chose to have home births instead of going to the hospital, and when I opted for corrective Lasik eye surgery instead of wearing prescription eyeglasses. Everyone thought of me as a pioneer about those choices, too, and they all worked out positively.

Dr. K's voice interrupted my misgivings and reinforced my trust. "Okay, Martha. Are you ready to start? We're going to establish your motor threshold with a few short pulses."

As soon as the chair reclined and I had full view of my feet, we were ready for take-off.

3,000 Pulses: Surviving Depression with TMS

"Yes—let's do this thing," I replied with a deep breath.

And so we began the set-up process for my TMS therapy.

"And how do you know you've got the right spot?" I asked, already wary that it might not work. "Will I feel anything and do I have to tell you when you've found it?"

"Your thumb will tell us!" they both said in unison.

Rosalind took my right hand and raised it so my elbow stayed on the cushion. She extended my thumb as if I were hitchhiking.

"We're going to begin by delivering single test pulses to the left side of your brain. We'll know we've connected with your motor strip when your right thumb moves with a little twitch."

They aligned my head with the machine's calibrated head positioning arms and recorded these head position settings that would be used for every session. Rosalind attached a paper tape across my forehead and connected it on both sides to the back of the headrest to hold my head in that now-determined place.

Dr. K lowered the curved apparatus holding the magnetic coil against my head. Suddenly I heard a little chime from the computer and a distinct, startling tapping sensation hit my scalp like a staple gun. Rosalind's eyes trained themselves on my right thumb as she waited for it to react to the pulse.

It didn't.

Dr. K moved the coil on my head slightly up and locked it in place again. Another chime followed by another pulse.

Nothing.

This process went on for several minutes with still no twitching in my hand or my thumb. My earlier worries reawakened as I fervently prayed it was the machine, the computer, or the technicians who needed adjustment, and not my brain's resistance to what I knew to be my last resort for wellness.

Echoes of admonitions to my childhood stubbornness surfaced as I conceded to Rosalind and the doctor, "Well, my family has always accused me of having a very hard head!"

They chuckled and once again assured me there was no

problem, and before long, after a few more hits from the coil, I felt a tiny tingle in my right hand. Another pulse—there—my ring finger twitched. Another pulse. Bingo! My thumb moved. We finally located the motor strip and now it was time to move the coil forward a few centimeters to find the exact location on my brain and figure out the adequate magnetic pulse intensity, or what they called "dosage".

Rosalind took my right arm and laid it down straight with my palm resting over the edge of the cushion. "Try to keep your wrist and hand as relaxed as possible."

As the doctor applied more single pulses at increasing strengths, Rosalind watched my fingers. At one point she held my hand loosely, still waiting to see—or at least feel—a twitching movement. The strength of the twitch would determine what percentage of magnetic pulse my brain should receive. Since I'd always been the kind of person who needs to know how things work—*How do they get the toothpaste in the tube?*—my fretfulness soon gave way to genuine fascination and curiosity.

The two women worked confidently, like a finely tuned machine as the computer chimed, the magnet tapped, Rosalind's head either shaking as a "no" or nodding as a "yes" while Dr. K input those responses into the computer and administered another exploratory pulse. Over a series of twenty responses, the computer captured the data, and through programmed algorithms in the system, it came up with the most effective dosage for my TMS standard motor threshold.

Once we were ready to begin the actual treatment, both Dr. K and Rosalind offered another welcoming dose of reassurance, reminding me I would eventually feel like a new person, with my depression relieved. Rosalind kindly but firmly reminded me that TMS is not a quick fix, and I should not expect to feel better until the fifteenth to twentieth session.

"Treatment response varies from patient to patient, and although it can take as long as twenty to thirty treatments to get results, what we've seen with our patients is ninety percent success."

"What happened to the ten percent who failed, and why didn't they succeed with TMS?"

Her response was quick and clear. "They gave up on the treatment, they lost patience, and they just weren't willing to wait for the stimulation to wake up their brains."

"Here's where my good old stubborn Irish genes come into play, I guess."

I rationalized that if I could withstand seventy hours of labor for my first child's birth without as much as an aspirin, I could certainly hang in here and get this done. If I could ride a commuter train five hours to New York City every day for twenty years, surely I can do this. If I could wake up every morning over the past many months wishing I would die and still be alive and sitting in this TMS chair, I can absolutely make the commitment to waiting twenty or so sessions for TMS to work its magic on me. I assumed a mantle of firm resolve and denounced any impatience that dared to interfere with my success.

With Dr. K's part of the process completed, she entrusted the remainder of the procedure to Rosalind, who offered me disposable earplugs to protect my ears from the magnetic pulse's loud tapping sound. She positioned another soft cushioned pad snuggly against the right side of my head in order to hold it firmly in place and for added comfort during the thirty-seven-minute treatment session.

"Would you like to listen to music or watch TV?" she asked.

At first I requested music, but the gentle piano and flutes in a New-Age CD hit a melancholy note within me, prompting more tears, so I quickly opted for the TV remote control. I made a good choice because the tapping sensation the machine delivered to my scalp was so intense I needed a full dose of distraction. I switched to the Travel Channel and sailed with the cameras on the Mediterranean to the Island of Crete. They swept me across the cloudless royal blue sky as we hovered over the Parthenon in

Athens. I'm sure the producers would've been delighted to know how their exotic segment on Greece transported me out of the unnerving experience I knew I'd have to tolerate every day for the next six weeks.

Here's how the treatment played out:

The computer announced the impending four seconds of pulsing with a chime similar to the "You've got mail" alert on a PC. I appreciated the warning, for no other reason than to brace myself for what felt like two hundred noogies on my head. In reality, it was forty pulses, and they happened at lightning speed, but despite the hard head I thought I had, they hurt. The twenty-six seconds of rest in between the pulsing action provided breathing room. I associated these intervals with the resting time I experienced between labor contractions during childbirth. I counted the seconds in between each warning chime and girded myself for the next round of hits. Four seconds on, twenty-six seconds off—on and off, on and off—until we reached three thousand pulses in a thirty-seven-and-a-half-minute session.

All the while Rosalind monitored me with a watchful eye through the window between the treatment room and her adjoining office. She also had a duplicate computer at her desk providing her with accurate readings of timing and position of the pulse to make sure the magnet maintained connectivity to the correct spot on my head.

Periodically she inquired, "Are you feeling okay?" to which I answered, "Yes, but this feels like a woodpecker having a temper tantrum on my head!"

"I know, it's uncomfortable to begin with, but you'll get used to it," she consoled me. With that she added it would eventually feel like more of an annoying sensation rather than pain. I wanted to believe her, but my inability to suck it up and deal with this initial discomfort needed more than just her reassuring words.

I decided to take the same approach as with a new pair of shoes. I thought about how, after a couple of weeks of regular wearing they eventually stretch out, conform to your feet, and you forget the pain it took to break them in.

Miraculously, they sometimes become your favorite pair.

12 | CASCO STREET REVISITED

"There is nothing like returning to a place that remains unchanged to find the ways in which you yourself have altered."

– Nelson Mandela

The TMS computer made its final chime after thirty-seven minutes of brain tapping.

"You're all done for today, Martha—you've done really well," Rosalind said.

She helped me out of the chair and reminded me, "I'll see you tomorrow at the same time, alright? And it won't take as long because now we've got your motor threshold all set up so you just have to come in, sit down, and have your treatment."

I left the TMS suite thankful I got through the first treatment so easily. I didn't feel tired, dizzy, or nauseated, and despite my whining about the discomfort, I didn't have the slightest hint of a headache.

Katherine and I walked in silence until we reached the car.

"Well, how do you feel? What was it like?" Her eyes searched my face for any signs of distress.

"It was like a trip to another planet." I paused and slowly shook my head, still processing what had actually occurred.

"It was peaceful, not as scary as I expected. Kind of surreal because I couldn't actually see anything happening. I just sat there and watched TV and let the machine tap on my head. I can't believe it was so simple."

The build-up to this day had been so dramatic, so fraught

with anticipation and anxiety. Now it felt almost anticlimactic.

The truth was, I felt extraordinary relief. I became inexplicably aware that I was standing in the past, present, and future—all in the same moment. As if the past's sadness and burdens melted into the present's relief that awakened a futuristic optimism in me. I felt a little smugness, as if I'd been inducted into a special society few people knew about. The only rules for membership were commitment to show up in Hartford every day, sit in a comfortable spa chair, and surrender my brain to invisible forces—magical magnetic pulses designed to re-enlist my inactive cerebral neurons, pulses that would deliver energy for the neurotransmitters I desperately needed to feel normal and happy.

"Why don't you let me drive your car so you can relax," Katherine offered. She commandeered the steering wheel and I gratefully tucked myself into the passenger seat belt.

We pulled out of the parking lot and immediately confused ourselves when we reversed the printed directions that brought us to Hartford. The usually reliable GPS incessantly admonished us with her singsong voice, "Recalculating". We turned left. "Recalculating." We turned right. "Recalculating." We were going nowhere fast.

"Just stay straight for a few blocks and maybe we can find a sign for I-84 up ahead," I suggested.

When we came to a vaguely familiar intersection, I sat up in my seat and blinked twice. The red traffic light gave me time to notice a granite tombstone-sized marker in the middle of a small grassy patch. I eyed the words "Welcome to Barry Square" chiseled into the gray stone.

"Katherine, you're not going to believe this, but we're sitting at the epicenter of my childhood. This is the neighborhood where I was baptized, went to grammar school, and where I lived until I was twelve!"

My childhood excursions in Hartford fifty years ago rarely

took me beyond Barry Square where we now sat frozen in time and place, waiting for a green light. Everything important resided in Barry Square—the library, the movie theatre, and the church.

Saint Augustine Roman Catholic Church towered ominously to my left with the priests' rectory right next to it. I could hardly believe my eyes—here it sat all those years, not even two blocks from Hartford Hospital. It seemed illogical that the non-Catholic hospital should be so close to Saint Augustine's, especially since, growing up in my strictly Roman Catholic world, the only hospital I knew was Saint Francis Hospital, ironically located way over on the other side of the city.

Hartford Hospital is where the "other people," the non-Catholics, went. Anything medical required the Catholic intercession only Saint Francis could provide: my younger siblings' births, the split chin requiring umpteen stitches when I fell down the cellar stairs at age two, my tonsillectomy at age eight, the trip to the emergency room for my sprained ankle—all were attended to through the grace of God at Saint Francis Hospital.

As if a time warp suddenly engulfed me, memories of Saint Augustine Church that I'd assumed were long forgotten flooded my mind and I felt helpless to stem the tide.

In that mausoleum of a church, at age seven I received my First Holy Communion wearing a lacy white dress accented with little pearls and a miniature tulle veil my mother sewed for me. All the girls wore white to signify our purity as recipients of "the Body of Christ". I recalled the tasteless, weightless Communion wafer placed ceremoniously on my extended tongue by the priest's enormous hand. Did the Holy Eucharist stick in the back of my throat and cause me to gag because I was so intimidated and anxiety-ridden, or was it such a dry little morsel that only a healthy swig of unattainable milk would release its grip on my palate?

At age eleven, when I was old enough to receive the sacrament of Confirmation, I officially became a "Soldier in Christ's Army," and the bishop slapped my cheek with his heavy, mutton-like hand to symbolically finalize the induction.

My most shocking memory flashed before my eyes—Monsignor Mulcahey's funeral. The nuns paraded the Saint Augustine School students from just a few blocks away into the church and past the bier displaying his dead body. We were expected to touch his cold hand and genuflect in silent veneration. I had never seen a dead person before and it horrified me. I wondered why they wanted us to touch a dead priest since we were forbidden to touch a living one. When I dared to glance at the corpse's face, all I noticed was a sinister black line defining the space between his upper and lower lips and curving menacingly downward at the corners. The sensation of his waxy, deadened skin permanently seared itself in my seven-year-old mind.

Suddenly my trip to Planet TMS morphed into a trip down Memory Lane.

"Well, this is no minor coincidence. How does it make you feel?" Katherine asked.

My always-the-introspective friend needed only to observe my wide-eyed, stunned expression and take my shaking hand in hers for an answer.

"I'm stunned. When we left Hartford and moved to Florida, I was twelve years old and I never, ever wanted to come back here again." All my senses tingled inside me. I stared at the cold stone façade of the building, past the enormous wooden doors and into the church's dark, shadowy interior where painted plaster statues of Jesus, Mary, and a legion of dead saints held court. I still smelled the ceremonial incense and melting candle wax lingering in every apse and pew. I remembered the sound of ghostly echoes reverberating throughout the massive space, giving startling voice to any unseen movement, real or imagined.

I didn't know whether to laugh or cry. "This is too goddamn ironic that I'm getting treated for depression within walking distance from where all my fears and anxiety started."

The traffic light cycled from red to green.

"Let's stay to the right and head down Maple Avenue. I want to go past Saint Augustine School and see if it's still standing," I said.

We drove three blocks as a slightly masochistic impulse rose within me, similar to rubber-necking to see a fatal car accident.

"Here, take a right at the next light on Clifford Street and pull over if—if you don't mind," I urged Katherine, who by now must have been wondering where this unplanned escapade was taking her.

There it stood as if the past fifty years never existed—Saint Augustine Catholic School. The distance from the church seemed so much shorter than how I remembered those many long, somber marches through the wet winter slush with forty other classmates. The nuns dutifully delivered us to the church from school for Masses, Confessions, and other religious ceremonies— any reason they could come up with to keep us in line—literally and figuratively. We marched single file, boys on one side, girls on the other, outfitted in the itchy wool maroon and gray uniform that branded us as obedient Catholic school children.

The exterior of the two-story building hadn't changed much. The yellow brick popularly used for construction back in the twenties retained its lifeless, utilitarian appearance. The windows and doors showed evidence of serious neglect, most likely due to lack of funds since the neighborhood itself reflected signs of a much poorer population. Broken windows were taped up with opaque plastic sheets. The fenced, blacktopped yard where we took recess and found our childhood friendships remained the same, only half as spacious as I remembered it.

"Have you had a long enough look?" Katherine nudged me.

"Yeah. I'm just remembering how scared I always felt behind those brick walls."

My parents decided the first four Pasternack kids would get their primary education at Saint Augustine Catholic School, not only with the three 'R's, but with every syllable of the irrefutable

Baltimore Catechism drilled into their little heathen heads. The nuns who taught us had their own cross to bear living in the patriarchal culture of the Catholic Church at that time. Their suppression was systematically transferred to their students whose primary desire was to get to heaven and learn multiplication tables in the bargain.

Not surprisingly, I couldn't ignore the feelings I failed to leave behind when we moved far away from Saint Augustine's to Florida in the early 1960s. I recalled my shame at being labeled a "bold, fresh girl" when I asked innocent questions that unwittingly contradicted the presiding nun's point of view. My persistent fear and insecurity came back to me that day, remembering how, at any moment, even the slightest misstep could sentence a child to the lonely, isolated cloakroom to serve a fifteen-minute punishment for speaking out of turn, inadvertently glancing at another student's paper, or not sitting up straight at one's desk. Bitter feelings surfaced—resentments of being suppressed and misunderstood by almost every nun who served as my teacher during the seven years I spent there. Sitting in my grown-up person's car, silently staring at this dilapidated, run-down hulk of a structure nearly fifty years later, anger simmered inside me and proved that my efforts to overcome these childhood issues had been in vain.

Unfortunately, my current depression only magnified their intensity. I felt indelibly stained with the rigors of my Catholic education, and even if any positive memories existed beyond my clouded vision, I had no mental or emotional capacity to entertain them at that moment.

I realized my propensity for perfectionism in everything I did thereafter could be, at least in part, attributed to the nuns and the Catholic Church. The nuns were perfection to me. They smelled of starched linen and soap. Their hands were soft and clean. They were Christ's brides and I wanted to be perfect like them. I wanted to do everything just right, look just right, and be every bit as right as the nuns wanted us to believe they were.

"You can take the child out of the Catholic school, Katherine, but you cannot take the Catholic school out of the child. Let's get out of here and drive the route I used to walk every day to school from my house on Casco Street."

Suddenly my motto of "the best way out is always through" flared up, and I hoped scratching this itch of morbid curiosity just might bring me to closure about what I now suspected were the beginnings of my lifetime's anxiety.

Katherine chauffeured me through Hartford's South End streets, past Sunshine Laundry where my dad pulled a meager weekly paycheck hauling other people's dirty clothes to support his growing brood. We passed the Campfield Avenue library where my mother tried so hard to get me to love reading despite my inability to concentrate, and over a half-mile along the avenue to 32 Casco Street at the edge of Goodwin Park. There our little white Cape Cod house still sat on the corner in a neighborhood long ago inhabited by like-minded Irish and Italian families with more than enough kids to go around.

I didn't see any signs of children now, and the tiny houses seemed cold and unfriendly even as they crowded in on each other. A small sign on our old front door warned, "Beware, attack dog on premises."

The subsequent owners had removed the picket fence my father single-handedly built one hot summer to corral us kids and protect us from the trucks barreling down South Street.

"It looks so small—how did my parents manage to fit all nine of us in it?" I asked myself in audible amazement. Two small bedrooms upstairs, one for the boys, the other for the girls; a living room, dining room, and a small den downstairs where my parents slept on a pull-out couch. Not even a finished basement to get us out of our mother's hair as she prepared vats of thrifty-minded suppers in her tiny kitchen.

The yard appeared completely inadequate for the many games

of tag and hide-and-seek we routinely played. But the spacious city park across the street provided us with what seemed like a country club: baseball diamonds; a public golf course; ponds for fishing in the summer and ice skating in the winter; and a playground where summertime activities included everything from arts and crafts to tap dancing lessons, swings, slides, and a basketball court.

The pièce de résistance came when the city of Hartford appropriated funds to install an Olympic-sized public swimming pool. I spent almost every hour of every summer day in that pool honing my competitive skills with swimming lessons, swim team practices, and water ballet routines. I had found something I was good at. I won swim meet medals and held a spot on the travel team. I could scull and pike better than any other girl in the synchronized swimming routines. I wanted to make my mark within a family where I felt invisible, for no other reason than the fact that I fell smack dab in the middle of the seven-kid line up. I never did make a name for myself in water sports, but the knowledge that I could do something out of the ordinary, better than someone else—and something none of my siblings did—helped to define me, although not necessarily for the best. I was evolving into a person who unknowingly had something to prove, and who would spend a lifetime working at it.

Katherine and I completed the pilgrimage to my old neighborhood with a long sigh and a final goodbye. Revisiting the places where I came from and how they fit into my current mental state gave me plenty to think about as we found our way homeward. Superficially, what life presented so long ago should have served up a healthy, emotionally balanced adult. I had a loving family with parents who provided a stable home in a wonderful neighborhood next to an idyllic park. Although it was a strict environment, I did get a solid education from those soapy nuns—after all, how many people did I know now who could actually diagram a sentence the way I could? And yes, seven children in a tight space lent itself to a certain amount of chaos, but it was organized chaos. And I always knew I was loved and would always be cared for in every sense of the word. But revisiting the past that day on Casco Street didn't alter how I felt about my current life.

Why, so many years later, did I continue to persist with thoughts that my life wasn't worth living? Where did the feelings of hopelessness and sadness come from? There was no denying that parents and teachers alike did the best they could to provide me with a decent upbringing. I relied on this rationalization to soothe my emotional wounds of always feeling different and separate from others.

Many years of talk therapy had also shed a certain amount of light on the issues usually attributed to depression and provided me with some relief, but my existing depressive state continued to erode me physically. I barely functioned day to day. My sleep, appetite, energy, memory, and concentration were shot to hell and I feared they'd never be restored.

Perhaps my hankering for answers would be met if, and when, TMS succeeded in restoring my life to normalcy. As Katherine and I sped down the interstate toward home, I methodically began planning the next day's four-hour round trip back to Hartford for my second TMS treatment.

Tomorrow, I'll make sure I get the directions right.

I didn't need another detour to my past. I wanted a clear route to my future.

13 | Two Down, Twenty-eight to Go

"When we are sure that we are on the right road, there is no need to plan our journey too far ahead; no need to burden ourselves with doubts and fears ... We cannot take more than one step at a time."

– Orison Swett Marden (1850-1924)

My right hand trembled as I stood in front of the mirror angling a mascara wand to my weepy eyes. The I-really-hope-this-TMS-thing-works jitters had set in since my return home the day before, and the alarm clock's ring so early that morning got my mind buzzing even more. Up until now, I usually awoke with no action plan, other than a vague approach to getting through another day without ending up in an emotional pit.

This morning's regimen reminded me of my days working at a real job for a real ad agency as a real professional. Now that I'd committed to doing six weeks of TMS treatments, I couldn't just roll out of bed—if and when the spirit moved me—to muddle my way through another pointless day, as I had been doing for almost a year. Even if I didn't feel like a normal person in a normal world, now I had to at least act like one.

Suddenly I had the proverbial "places to go, people to meet, things to do" happening again. Finding the fastest, most efficient route and arriving on time for my appointment, having enough gas in the car, and making sure I remembered any and all important details—the pressure ran through my head like the news crawl in Times Square.

I gave myself extra time to start the video and written journal

I decided to keep during my six weeks of TMS. I had tried journaling a few times in the past but never stuck to it. When I'd reread my entries, I always thought they smacked of self-indulgence and pettiness and I'd cringe with self-judgment. But since I'd challenged the insurance company so fiercely, I wanted to be sure I kept tabs on my progress. I sat down in front of the monitor, switched on my computer and adjusted the little eyeball camera attached to the screen.

"Ahem, uh, it's Tuesday, May 4, 2009, and this is my second day of TMS treatment. I'm a little nervous, but I want to record how I am today, which is pretty awful, but hopefully I'll look a lot better in a few weeks after I finish the treatments."

It seemed awkward talking to myself, especially since I hardly knew how I felt or what to say. I stopped the camera after just a few minutes, feeling rather foolish about the whole thing, but unconsciously I knew TMS was enough of an offbeat therapy that others might not believe me if it really worked. I wanted to have something tangible to prove to others—but mainly to the insurance company that they hadn't wasted their money on me. The old saying "The proof is in the pudding" came to mind. I was the pudding, and I hoped the daily journal would be my proof.

As I closed the front door behind me, Josie cocked her head and eyed me through the front window with a "Where are you going?" look. We were quite a pair, spending our uneventful days together, hardly ever venturing out. I fretted over whether she could handle the adjustment of being alone every day for the next six weeks, just as I wondered if I would be able to manage the long, monotonous car rides.

Echoes of Rosalind's warnings—"This isn't a quick fix. Don't expect to feel anything different for at least a couple of weeks"—served as a reminder to hold my expectations in check and prepare for the long haul, figuratively and literally. I loaded myself into the car, praying for strength to keep going. I couldn't help but notice how truly scared and alone I felt, despite the many loving supporters encouraging me as I pursued this nontraditional path.

At first I wondered if I should make the trip alone every day. John, my sisters, and dear friends all offered to drive me, but since I didn't feel any side effects at all from my first treatment, I felt confident I could manage on my own. As I craned my neck and backed the car out of the driveway, I considered that a daily travel companion might distract me from any negative thoughts. But the energy it would take to politely keep up a conversation for the long car ride ended my internal debate. No, I concluded, this gig was mine, and mine alone. I thought to myself, "This is very similar to birthing a baby. No matter how many attendants plant themselves at her bedside, the bottom line is it's the woman who's doing the labor and it's the woman who's pushing that baby out." After my children were born, my response to "Who delivered your baby?" seemed pretty obvious to me: "I delivered my baby—I'm the one who did all the work! Dr. So-and-So just caught the baby!"

Following that little pep talk of self-empowerment and a couple of miles down the country roads leading me away from my house, I gave the gas pedal a heavy foot as I climbed the ramp onto the highway.

∿

Unlike the previously gloomy day, the sun showed up that morning. Grateful to have its company, my ninety-minute drive proved to be uneventful and my fears of being late unnecessary. The route I chose brought me to the exit where the state capitol building and government offices ceremoniously sat. I carefully navigated through the unfamiliar city streets, past the state supreme court and a variety of other municipal buildings. Female attorneys congregating outside the courthouse in their smart suits clutched legal files as if they were teddy bears. I noticed how disenfranchised I had become from a normal life. How I missed the days when I wore fashionable business clothes to meetings, where critical business problems required my once-sought-after business savvy. Between the disastrous crisis of the drug and alcohol overdose and then losing my job, I couldn't help feeling like a complete loser.

My identity clung so dearly to my job; unemployment left me rudderless. Pangs of wishing I could again be a part of something bigger than myself welled up inside me—something that mattered to others, and something to dispel the isolation my depressive world had degenerated into. With a sigh of combined rationalization and anemic hope, I silently conceded, I guess this is my normal for the time being. TMS could mean being a part of something bigger than myself, and even if it only matters to me and my little world, that'll have to be okay for now.

A few city blocks later, "Carmine of the Garmin GPS" guided me with her attentive voice into the parking lot of the Hartford Hospital Institute of Living. The bright sun and fresh spring air washed my face and revived me from the long car ride's trance. I entered the treatment area where Rosalind met me, and I couldn't help but notice patients with dazed looks on their faces, staring blankly at their laps or vacantly into thin air. Some were propped up on stretchers, others slumped in wheelchairs.

"What are all these people waiting for?" I whispered as we filed past them on our way to her office.

She replied in one breath without skipping a beat. "Oh, those are ECT patients recovering from their treatment. Are you ready for Day Two?"

"Uh, yes." I quickly followed her into the TMS room as I edged myself around an orderly jockeying one of the patients out the door into a waiting mini-ambulance. I felt pity for the folks in the hallway, and I wondered if it was really the aftereffects of their ECT treatment or their extreme illness that left them so lifeless. *God, I'm so grateful I can drive myself to and from these treatments.*

Rosalind collected my watch and earrings in the pretty china dish out of the TMS magnet's range. I took my place in the treatment chair and prepared for the intense tapping. While she carefully positioned the magnetic coil and dialed up the computer settings, I meekly complained of the tenderness I experienced on my scalp during yesterday's treatment.

"I hope I can get through this today. It really hurt my head yesterday, even after I took the two Tylenol Dr. K recommended."

"I can adjust the coil a little bit to make you more comfortable," she offered. She moved the coil a little higher on my head, away from my temple, and gave me a test pulse. "How's that?"

"Pretty good, still maybe a little too close to my temple."

Rosalind adjusted the coil's position two more times with test pulses and we finally found a tolerable spot higher on my head. I didn't want her to think me a fussy patient with my complaining, but I also didn't want my inability to deal with the tapping to cause me to wimp out and not come for treatments. I was glad I spoke up and even happier she could accommodate me by finding a less sensitive target further away from my left temple. I settled in. Earplugs in place, TV remote in hand, I squared my jaw and signaled, "I'm good to go."

After a few minutes into my session, Rosalind's watchful eye through the window between her office and the TMS room caught me weeping. She entered with a box of tissues and a dose of much needed encouragement. Despite our earlier efforts to move the coil, I still hadn't adjusted to the intensity of the pulsing, the immediate reason for my tears. Everything under the sun bothered me, even when I knew it shouldn't. The depression made me so sensitive that even a foot massage irritated me. I yearned to be normal like everyone else, and I wished I didn't have to work so damned hard to stay alive.

"I'm sorry to be such a baby about this," I whimpered through a handful of tissues. "Maybe it's because I feel so vulnerable and fragile."

"You are going to get used to the sensation, I promise you," she vowed. "If you don't get used to it in a few days, I'll eat a bowl of worms."

We both laughed as she stood with me for the next few series of pulses. I began to feel more relaxed and surmised my tenseness probably contributed to the pain level. *Nothing goes well when you're tense, Martha, you know that. Chill.*

Within a few minutes I recognized myself as the self-appointed guest of honor at my own pity party. With a final sniffle, I simply resigned myself to the next half-hour's tapping, knowing I had no choice but to tough it out.

The time passed only as quickly as I could escape into the TV's mindless distraction. Because I couldn't see the computer screen sitting behind my left shoulder displaying the status of my session, and my watch was on the far table—a protective distance from the machine's magnet—I had no idea where we were in the scheme of the thirty-seven-and-a-half-minute session. With my head held firmly in place on the left side by the TMS coil and counterbalanced on the right side with the smaller pad for stability, even a peek at progress achieved versus time remaining wasn't an option.

My previous business experience had focused on operations, efficiency, and project management, so naturally I soon devised a way of tracking the time. I remembered that most TV shows are programmed for approximately nine minutes of entertainment and then three to four minutes of commercials. I took note of when the show started and when the ads played and added up the minutes. This strategy became a great way to pass the time and safeguarded me from becoming an impatient patient. Before long, any teary despondency disappeared into relaxation as the Food Network's feature on trussing a chicken captured my undivided attention, along with the intermittent commercials that provided me with time markers.

The next time Rosalind came into the room wasn't to cheer

me. "Time's up!" she chirped and gently helped me out of the chair. As I reattached my jewelry and started to bid her goodbye until the next day, she asked, "Wait, do you have time to meet with our research assistant for a few minutes?"

"Oh, what for?" I responded somewhat cautiously. I wondered, "Do I have a bigger problem than I thought and the researchers need to take a closer look at me?"

"It will only take about a half-hour. We're keeping Hamilton Depression Rating Scales for our patients so we can track their status when they begin TMS and then follow their progress throughout the course of treatment and for several months afterward."

Susan, my talk therapist, had mentioned these scores during our work together almost a year ago, so I was somewhat familiar with them. To my knowledge, however, I had never been assessed. The idea that I could have a measuring tool for TMS's efficacy appealed to my sense of order and accountability.

"Sure," I nodded. "I've got plenty of time."

I gathered my belongings and headed to the waiting room where a young woman greeted me with a quiet smile. Her short, neatly styled dark hair matched her firm handshake.

"Mrs. Rhodes? I'm Keera. I'm a research assistant here at Hartford Hospital and I'd like to ask you a few questions that won't take too long."

We crossed the hall to a stark, unoccupied office where I sat in a rigid wooden chair as she took her place in another facing me. The overhead fluorescent lighting didn't do my vanity any favors. The room was cold with scant, mismatched furnishings. It felt more like an interrogation room at the local police station.

The Hamilton Depression Rating Scale, also known as HAM-D, is a series of twenty-one questions clinicians use to determine a patient's level of depression. The process is quite simple, designed to rank severity of depression symptoms pertaining to physical and behavioral areas such as mood, sleep patterns, and appetite, among others. All that's required is for the patient to orally respond to the questions. The good news for me: there were no wrong answers. All I had to do was tell the truth—if only I could pinpoint the truth, considering my mind's foggy state.

Tall, thin, pretty, soft-spoken with a spirit to match, Keera personified objectivity. As she queried me about my diet, energy, libido, and any ideations for self-destruction, I wrestled with trying to answer her questions honestly and accurately. I wanted my answers to tell the truth now so when I felt happy again, just like my journal, I'd have proof that TMS worked.

"Have you been able to fall asleep in a reasonable amount of time in the past week?"

"Yes. I could sleep sixteen hours a day if I didn't feel so guilty about it," I answered.

"Have you unintentionally lost or gained any weight in the past week?"

"No. Not unless you count the extra forty pounds I put on since I started taking antidepressants."

"Have you had any thoughts of suicide in the past week?"

"No, not of actually committing suicide. I already proved I couldn't do that successfully. But if a doctor told me I had terminal cancer, I'd thank him, go home, and do nothing."

The exercise seemed simple enough. I answered yes or no, or as Keera discerned from my more elaborate replies, she rated them one to four. The questions were straightforward and benign, but my responses felt complicated and almost malignant to me. The words choked like a piece of dry bread when the truth of how miserable I felt passed from my lips onto her clipboard. My chest tightened and I stifled threatening emotional spasms. The pathetic reality of my existence no longer remained inside my head. Now it was defined in neat rows of check-marked boxes on Keera's HAM-D form. I didn't want to break down in front of this sweet young woman whose only reason for being with me was to gather information. I doubted she had even a tissue to spare me.

She must have sensed my struggle because she kept repeating, "I'm sorry I have to ask you the same kind of questions over and over. We're putting your answers anonymously into a database to share TMS results with other hospitals and universities, so it's important that we get through this."

I quietly assured her, "No, no, don't apologize, it's okay with me, really," and lamely offered, "I support any research the hospital wants to do." I buoyed my attitude by reasoning that if this disabling curse of mine could do any bit of good for someone's research project, then hats off to all of us.

Rosalind's prediction of how long the interview would take proved to be true. Less than thirty minutes later, Keera and I finished our Q&A and we agreed to meet once every other week for the remainder of my treatment period, plus once a month by telephone for a year thereafter. I liked her, and I liked the fact that I could contribute to someone else's efforts.

Mission almost accomplished, I drove home wondering if and when I would feel less depressed, cautiously disallowing premature and unfettered optimism. When I finally pulled into the driveway, I made a beeline to the couch where a nap would seal the deal on what now looked like a rather productive day. After all, I had managed to organize myself sufficiently to get to Hartford on time—alone. I made it through another session of intense tapping without wimping out, even though I did cry a little bit. I met with a total stranger and responded to her battery of very personal questions, even if I couldn't be sure of my accuracy. And for the most part I managed to minimize my tears, at least while driving on the interstate.

Although I was physically exhausted, for the first time in months a vaguely familiar feeling of accomplishment settled over me. "Two sessions down, twenty-eight to go," I sighed. I stretched out, closed my eyes, and warmed myself in the late afternoon sun pouring through the family room window. Josie snuggled in alongside me, offering her vote of confidence with an occasional lick on my free hand as I gratefully stroked her soft coat with the other.

14 | PART-TIME JOB—FULL-TIME COMMITMENT

*It's Friday, May fourteenth. I'm just so tired. I wake up
and tell myself to just get through the day. Try to stay
positive, try to have hope, and if I can't have hope, at
least don't have despair.*

— My Video Journal Entry

Two weeks crawled by. Ten days of driving to Hartford for
sessions lasting less than half the time it took me to get there.
I still awoke every morning with a foreboding that reminded me
of the movie *Groundhog Day*—in which every day begins in exactly
the same way. At least the routine's repetitive steps got me out
the door on schedule: breakfast, shower, find something cheerful
to wear, fix my hair, and apply makeup. Things I hadn't done
since I'd been unemployed. The routine kept me from losing
hope, however, and having a purpose with a goal comforted me. I
believed if I could play the tortoise's strategy of "slow and steady
wins the race," I had a decent chance of coming through this as
either win, place, or show—I didn't really care which, just as long
as I got through it.

"A watched pot never boils." That's an old saying my mom
pitched to us kids whenever we got antsy about waiting for
something. Her convoluted advice usually made me feel more
impatient than I felt to begin with, particularly because it didn't
make a hell of a lot of sense to my youthful logic. My smart ass
self always wanted to snipe back with, "Well then, turn up the
damn heat and make it boil!" When I caught myself obsessing
over whether or not TMS was having an effect, I heard Mom

chiming in from the grave and I gave it a second, more adult listen. Yeah, maybe I just need to surrender to this process and be patient. I hoped she knew how much her advice meant to me thirteen years after she'd passed away.

Rosalind and Dr. K didn't have any advice for me about the long wait, other than the assurance that I would definitely notice the positive result of the treatment when it finally arrived. I figured that meant when I stopped waking up every morning with those dreadful feelings I described to my therapist as "emotional nausea."

When the weekends arrived I made every effort to avoid crying in front of John for fear of raising his doubts about my progress. But during the weekdays while he was at work, I just couldn't help myself. I felt utterly useless. I woke up exhausted with no energy to carry out the day's newly established routine. What inspired me to get out of bed, however, was everyone's expectation that I would faithfully make the journey to Hartford.

Yes, journey—not just any ordinary trip. Because the whole TMS effort was such a big deal, my imagination had assigned the daily drive to a much more significant category, something akin to a pilgrimage or odyssey. I knew I needed to temper this overly dramatic point of view. I decided to put TMS therapy in a relatable context to give it a more down-to-earth perspective— TMS therapy became my new job.

During my early days working in advertising, I served as a temporary mechanical artist and back-end art director for several small New York agencies who couldn't afford full-time staff. It was a common practice in the industry to use freelance help, especially when clients' needs were either fleeting or unpredictable. I became very successful in the ad business as a reliable resource for this ever-present demand. The hiring managers could always count on Martha Rhodes to show up on time, do a great job, and give them an honest day's work. Sometimes those days turned into weeks and months, providing my young family with some healthy paychecks. I reaped the financial benefits, and the agency had my solid commitment for however long they needed a workhorse such as myself.

It occurred to me that by holding the six weeks of TMS in the same context as I had with those freelance gigs, I could maintain the necessary stamina for what promised to be a lengthy process. As a freelancer, I never became too attached to the agency or the people in it, because I knew I'd be leaving at some point. The freelance agreement obviated any long-term worries about worker relationships, commuter challenges, or career decisions. It was all about the project at hand, with a beginning and end date. This current situation had similar characteristics: long daily commute, six-week project or, rather, treatment plan, show up on time, and get the job done. No problem. So every morning, just as I had done when I had a real job, I packed up a nice little lunch and coffee-to-go cup and got myself to my TMS treatment as unfailingly as I had throughout my working career. It worked brilliantly—I gave myself a part-time job with a sense of purpose that afforded me much needed energy.

Now that I was getting out of bed earlier than I had in months, I continued to use the time to either write in my journal or videotape myself. Keeping a journal was new for me because, in the past, I thought it took valuable time I could never spare. I wrote with a stream of consciousness and without editing my entries. Talking to the video camera was more of a challenge, mainly because I looked so pained and pitiful and it insulted my vanity. But a little voice inside my head urged me to keep track of my days and I'm thankful I listened to it. Journaling allowed me to be myself with myself. I didn't worry about anyone else's impression of me, nor did I care if what I wrote mattered to anyone else. They were my thoughts and feelings, and mine alone. I eventually discovered that the daily writing exercise became an integral part of my healing process.

～

By the beginning of the third week, the reality of the boring three hours of driving set in. The excitement and anticipation of receiving TMS treatment no longer glowed within me. And while the depressed mood persisted, I tried not to obsess over the treatment's effect, or lack of it. In order to remain on track, I knew I had to come up with some sort of diversion, or the daily drill would wear me down.

My car's GPS device gave me a unique sense of control, particularly when road construction crews created miles-long traffic delays on I-84. Fortunately, I discovered the "detour" function on the gadget. On more than one occasion, as I headed for the nearest exit ramp at the first sign of trouble, a comforting smugness replaced the anxiety of being late for my appointment.

And thanks to the magic of my GPS companion, I was also free to switch up my travel route for scenic variety. I pushed myself. *Find other things to do while you're out and about, either before or after the trip to Hartford. Break up the routine and add a little fun to these six weeks.* Fun seemed an odd way to approach the whole thing, especially since fun had been missing from my life for so long.

One day during Week Three, after my TMS session I rerouted my return trip, hoping this might be, well, fun. I set my course to revisit the different areas in Hartford's South End where I grew up, chancing I would remember them a half-century later. I guess my anxiety-provoking first trip back in time with Katherine to visit my old grammar school had given me a desire to find some of the good memories, too.

My father knew the streets well. Dad would give Mom a break from the chaos in the tiny Casco Street house by taking anyone who wasn't in a baby carriage down to Franklin Avenue for a Lincoln Dairy ice cream cone. Other times for a special treat on a hot summer night, all of us kids squeezed into the powder blue 1954 Plymouth station wagon knee-to-knee and butt-to-butt, and he'd herd us over to the Berlin Turnpike for a drive-in movie.

Dad took us on a regular Friday night mission to a large

bakery warehouse down on Wethersfield Avenue for cheap bread. We'd wait for the trucks returning from their deliveries to back into a cavernous, open garage where they'd dump all sorts of day-old bread and leftover pastries onto an expansive wooden table.

Dad would line the team of us strategically around its perimeter and coach us.

"Keep an eye out for the pumpernickel, Michael!" or "Maria, grab two of those raisin breads!" We artfully ducked under elbows and snuck between grown-ups' legs, competing with them as they frantically pursued bargain bread for their own growing broods. Since our eyes barely cleared the lip of the table, my younger brother Vinnie and I claimed whatever fell to the floor as our contribution to the land grab.

I'm sure my mom was quite happy with whatever bread we could snag for the pennies it cost for our trouble. It took a hell of a lot of peanut butter and jelly sandwiches to feed seven kids on a laundry deliveryman's salary, but we never went hungry.

Most days after my TMS treatment, rather than hopping on the highway ramp close to the hospital, I usually preferred to drive out of Hartford past the church and the school and over to the perimeters of my old neighborhood. The three-story brick building that was once a casket company still stood on Maple Avenue. Since I'd never been to a funeral home, I thought this was where the dead people ended up before they were buried. Whenever I passed it on my way to and from school, I scurried along the sidewalk with my head bent down for fear of seeing resurrected cadavers peering at me out of its eerie dark windows. Now the once dirty bricks were sandblasted to their original bright red color, and large brass letters decorated the building's front. The casket company had morphed into the South End Senior Wellness Center. After fifty years I couldn't miss the irony, even if I tried. No longer a place for dead seniors—now they were saving them in there.

When I ran out of old familiar areas to revisit, I sometimes left the TMS center and satisfied an impulse to explore new areas of the city, reliving another childhood pastime.

My friend Elaine and I would deliberately ride our bikes into unknown surrounding neighborhoods, making random turns left and right down streets we'd never been on before. The game of "Let's Get Lost on Purpose" sharpened our sense of direction and thrilled us when we ultimately conquered our self-inflicted fear by instinctively finding our way back home. The boys got to ride their bikes anywhere they wanted, but we were restricted to our immediate neighborhood. So we made sure our mothers didn't know, which only added to the audacity of our escapades and inflated the notion that we were clever, intrepid explorers who could conquer the world. At the end of each adventure, Elaine and I would breathlessly congratulate each other with a promise to keep our shared secret.

I drew on the memory of those adventures to remind myself that I could find my way out of this depressingly lost place by holding fast to my instincts. The independence I knew I possessed at that young age fortified my faltering confidence in beating the depression that seemed to be increasing, not abating.

～

Around day twelve or thirteen during my third week, I noticed a marked decline in my mood. Everything around me felt gloomier and raw. When I showed up for my fourteenth treatment, I guardedly said to Rosalind, "I feel miserable. Have you had patients who feel worse before they get better with TMS?"

"No, not really. We have patients who complain of increased anxiety, but not worsened depression. I'll mention it to Dr. K so she knows what you're experiencing."

My heart plunged as low as my mood. I could easily understand someone having increased anxiety. After all, it is a tedious process, one that comes at a considerable expense, both financially and time-wise. But I wasn't feeling increased anxiety, because I wasn't expecting a quick turnaround—I fully understood from my preliminary meetings with Rosalind and Dr. K that TMS wasn't a quick fix. And since I had insurance coverage, I wasn't even worried about the money. But I didn't expect to feel worse than when I started.

For the next few trips back and forth to my appointments, I drove with a box of tissues in my lap. At times I had to pull the car off the road because the tears made it impossible to drive safely. I sobbed out loud, thankful to be alone where no one could hear me. "How could this be happening to me? I've done everything I'm supposed to do. I haven't skipped even a day. Oh, God, maybe this is never going to help me after all." My mind raced, groping for answers and pleading with the universe to let this be only a temporary setback.

Two days later as I got in the TMS chair, Rosalind said, "You know how you mentioned you felt worse the other day? The very next day, another patient who's a female and about your age complained of the same thing."

Relieved and secretly delighted, I wondered if this was a case of misery-loves-company on my part before I asked, "Really? Is she crying and worried TMS isn't working for her either?"

I was unsure if I should have been disappointed for the both of us or relieved that there might be a logical explanation. Rosalind assured me she and Dr. K were looking into the data. I needed an answer because I worried that my brain was being zapped in the wrong direction.

By my next appointment I had my answer. I learned that the reason for what I've come to refer to as "the Dip" is somewhat common and logical. Patients have reported the appearance of increased depression early in antidepressant treatment for more than fifty years. Most medical explanations agree that as neurotransmitter balance is restored during antidepressant therapy, the initial improvement is usually increased physical energy. However, a patient's mood can subsequently respond with a symptom of increased depressed feelings because his or her brain structure is undergoing a rebalancing. Some patients with depression may have underlying bipolar disorder, and the activation by antidepressant treatment (medications or stimulation) might lead to a worsening of mood. Many times this is temporary as it can be the brain's way of adapting to a new electrochemical balance.

In a nutshell, my brain was being reconfigured. The daily three thousand pulses reawakened it from its under-productive state, but my brain then needed to reset itself with the appropriate balance of neurotransmitters I required to feel good.

"It's always darkest before the dawn." I laughed to myself at how my mother's spirit lovingly nudged me when I recalled another of her famous quotes.

I related this homestretch challenge to my childbirth experience when, after interminable hours of labor, I reached what my Lamaze instructor warned me about—transition. Transition is generally the shortest phase of labor, but without a doubt, the most difficult. It's the fifteen to thirty minutes when the woman is the most emotionally needy and wants to give up. She's apt to cry out, "I can't do this and I want to go home!" Getting through transition means that the painful contractions have done their job and have fully dilated the cervix to ten centimeters so the baby can enter the birth canal. If a woman pushes before getting through transition, her baby can't pass through and the mother is wasting her energy trying to push. She needs to stay focused on handling the contractions that will open the cervix for her baby. It's only then that the midwife or doctor says, "Push!"

Even though I wondered if I should give up on TMS— and I doubted I could go another day feeling so depressed—I felt grateful to have had my childbirth transition experience to associate this emotional dip. I accepted I was in TMS transition and simply needed to concentrate on the process of day-to-day treatments to get through. I was rebirthing myself. I convinced myself that I would soon be ready to bear down and "Push!"

"A watched pot never boils, Martha."

Okay, Mom, okay—I finally get it.

15 | THE LIFT

Monday, May twenty-third. I feel different, less of an aching in my heart. Maybe TMS is working. I don't want to get too excited though. I'm afraid I'll jinx it.

— My Video Journal Entry

It happened to me many times during those strenuous work and commuter years. My eyelids opened halfway, I'd glance at the alarm clock and rustle my body to start my "gotta get up and go" engine. Just as the gears began churning in my head, I'd realize in surprised relief, "Oh, wow, it's not Friday, it's Saturday—and I don't have to go to work. I can go back to sleep. Yes!"

This happened to me at the end of my third week of TMS treatment, and directly on the heels of "the Dip." I awoke on Saturday morning with a feeling similar to those previous weekday-weekend mix-ups, when I reminded myself, *Oh, it's Saturday—no TMS today.* But the old "Oh, wow" and "Yes!" moments didn't pop up, even though I was glad not to have to make the long trip.

I lay there for a moment—very still, only half-awake. *Something's missing here. What's different about this morning?* The brightest sunlight I'd seen in what seemed like years flooded the room. I blinked my eyes once or twice, peeked over the hem of the fluffy comforter, and suddenly realized, *It's gone.* The dreadful emotional nausea that choked me every morning was missing. *I feel ... different. Am I dreaming, or is this real?*

Quietly, without any mental fanfare, I sat up, gingerly stretched, and swung my legs over the bedside. A distinct lightness accompanied me from the bedroom to the bathroom sink. My reflection in the mirror looked disappointingly the same as it had for the past year and a half—wan and wrinkled with puffy bags under my tired eyes. The cold water I splashed on my face failed to improve it. I stared intently at myself in the mirror, however, because I knew that internally my mind felt calmer, lighter, uncluttered—just different.

Could I actually be feeling better? I searched my eyes for what felt like a full minute, waiting to see if any sad emotions would well up in them under the scrutiny. No tears. No anxiousness or agitation. Just a subtle—but undeniable—easiness. I made my way to the kitchen. Perhaps a cup of strong coffee would put things in a realistic perspective.

"Good morning, sweetie. How're you feeling today?" John asked as he sipped his second cup. As usual, he was up and dressed before me, and as cheerful a person anyone could hope to start a day with.

I honestly didn't know how to respond to his well-meaning question. I hesitated to prematurely blurt out, "I'm terrific. I'm cured. The depression is gone. TMS is working." What if I just wanted it to work so badly that my mind resorted to imagining it worked? Could this just be a rebound from "the Dip" and part of a perpetual roller-coaster ride of ups and downs?

During our initial consultation, Dr. K explained how some of her patients described their success with TMS as an "Aha moment"—a sudden feeling of an emotional cloud lifting. This didn't feel too "Aha" to me. It felt more like a nudge, a little sniff of fresh air coming through the trees, a distant tune I could barely hear, but longed to sing. Nothing definite, but nevertheless unmistakably present—temporarily or otherwise. The previous week's decline in my mood landed me in such an abyss that I wondered if I'd be able to recognize my own eureka moment—if and when it arrived—so I kept this mysterious development to myself. If I had misread the signs of improvement, I didn't want to put John through the ordeal of cleaning up the fallout of my disillusionment.

By the following Monday morning, however, my brighter, less encumbered attitude surpassed my weekend's cautious optimism. I could feel the lightness Dr. K described. It was subtle, but indisputable. I didn't feel the ever-present burden of suppressing tears, nor did I need to summon the superhuman strength it previously took to appear upbeat. On the other hand, I wasn't experiencing an emotional high either. Instead of diving into a huge ocean wave all at once, it felt like I was standing on the shore letting the waves lap my feet, then my calves, then my thighs, until I felt accustomed to the water's temperature, and then submerged my entire body.

During the commute to Hartford throughout that next, fourth week, I felt myself gradually feeling happier. My awareness of how the little things in life were changing tipped me off that TMS was doing its job. Where I usually spent the ninety minutes' drive in gloomy silence, I now listened to music on the car's CD player. As the days moved on, my music selections progressed from light jazz, to lively folk rock, and then to robust Broadway show tunes. At one point I laughingly caught myself bellowing out the title song of *Hello, Dolly!* as I slipped the car in and out of the semi-trucks' caravans with the confidence of a Mario Andretti.

Now my post-treatment excursions assumed a more positive tone. The doleful, regretful feelings haunting me about my childhood transformed into more upbeat, tender recollections. My diversion *du jour* near the end of my six-week tour took me to the Berlin Turnpike in Wethersfield.

One of the very first McDonald's restaurants in the country debuted on the Berlin Turnpike back in the 1950s. All of us kids squeezed into the Plymouth station wagon, excited. Although our dad didn't have the extra money for the burgers, we wanted to see what this new attraction was all about. At that time only an abbreviated golden arch distinguished its less than ubiquitous brand, along with wide red and white horizontal stripes on the building's exterior. Mouthwatering aromas wafting from the little fast food stand teased all our senses as we drove through the parking lot with our curious tongues hanging out.

Fifty years and millions of Quarter Pounders later—there it stood. I pulled into the drive-thru lane of the very same, but new and improved, McDonald's Playland extravaganza and rolled down my car window. A tinny voice greeted me from a speaker embedded in the drive-thru menu board.

"Welcome to McDonald's. May I take your order, please?"

I leaned my head out the door and surprised myself with my request.

"I'd like a Happy Meal." I mentally transformed myself into a six-year-old as I relived this unfulfilled childhood memory.

"Will there be anything else?" The garbled voice waited while I reconsidered.

"Nope. That's it. Just one Happy Meal, please."

"Hamburger, cheeseburger, or McNuggets?"

"Um, hamburger, please, with soda."

"That will be two-eighty-nine. Please pay at the next window."

I instinctively worried if I'd broken an unwritten McDonald's law by ordering a Happy Meal as an adult. *I hope they'll give it to me—I wonder if grown-ups are allowed to have Happy Meals without proof of a hungry child.* I edged the car forward to the pick-up window and waited only a minute before the glass panel slid to the side.

A long arm extended a neat little box plastered with Ronald McDonald's broad smile. I quickly swapped it for three dollars and drove away before taking my eleven cents change. I smiled to myself as I fumbled to open the little box. A miniature Mermaid Barbie sat atop the pint-sized burger neatly tucked in with a soda and French fries.

I shook my head in amazement and laughed to myself. "God, we would've killed for one of these when we were kids."

∿

"The Lift" redefined everything in my life. I began to answer the telephone on the first or second ring, and I returned calls that friends and family left on the answering machine. I started reading entertaining novels again instead of poring over self-help books that only magnified my personal shortcomings. John and I went to the movies where I laughed and cried along with the rest of the audience. Our house needed a thorough cleaning after so many months of sore neglect, and I felt strong enough to tackle the more challenging jobs like cleaning the refrigerator and reorganizing kitchen cabinets. The day the iron and ironing board came out, I felt sure I had turned a corner with TMS.

Keera and I continued to track my HAM-D ratings once a week after the TMS treatment. My previously teary sessions answering simple questions now took on a much easier, less tortured dynamic. When we first met, my scale numbers climbed as high as twenty-eight. They began their happy descent to single digits somewhere into the fourth week of treatments until I ultimately reached an astonishing zero on the scale—total remission from depressive symptoms.

Life at home, life with family and friends—and life in general—became wonderfully manageable. I no longer flew off the handle when I forgot where I put my car keys. I sensed John's relief when we went to restaurants and I didn't find fault with a hapless waiter. Nevertheless, it took patience to get through the TMS process, but the beauty of it lay in how seamlessly I transitioned from depression to good health. I felt comfortable maintaining my "slow and steady wins the race" game plan. The subtle, gradual improvement bolstered my confidence that my re-engineered mental health would not be misconstrued as a manic high or a brief interlude before another round of despair set in. My TMS mojo was finally working. That's all I needed to know.

As the final week of treatment drew near, my trips to Hartford seemed to get shorter. I had to admit to myself and to Rosalind on my final treatment day, "I don't want to stop coming here. I'm going to miss everyone at the TMS center, I'm going to miss the routine, and I'm actually going to miss the car rides."

Dr. K came into the room to say goodbye and congratulate me on my recovery.

"I'd still like you to come for treatments for the next three weeks but not every day. Come Monday, Wednesday, and Friday the first week, then Tuesday and Thursday the following week, and only once the last week, whatever day works for you. This way you'll ease off of the treatments."

"After I finish that, should I come back for maintenance treatments?" I asked.

"You'll want to keep doing your journal and be mindful if you start to feel depressed, but you've responded so well to TMS I doubt you'll have to worry too much about maintenance right now," she assured me.

Prior to FDA approval, clinical trials utilized this titration paradigm to gradually taper treatment and theoretically reduce a rebound into depression, so Dr. K held to the practice.

On my last day in Hartford, I felt happier and healthier than I had in years. My whole demeanor changed from slow, sluggish, and frail to energized, optimistic, and strong. I felt a little sad to be leaving Rosalind and Dr. K's weekly care, wondering what I'd do with my days now that my part-time TMS gig—my freelance summer job—was ended. On the other hand, I felt like a total success and ready to face a new world no longer shrouded with a heavy mantle of dread draped over every heartbeat. I crossed my fingers that the TMS effect would hold, but I resolved that I would come back for more sessions if even an inkling of depression returned.

∽

Sometime during July or August, several weeks after I completed my last session, John and I attended a friend's theatre performance in a production at Yale University. After the show she invited us to join several cast members whom we didn't know for a post-theatre celebration. At first I didn't want to go, concerned I wouldn't be able to keep up a conversation with so many new people.

The pub-like restaurant was noisy and overcrowded. I looked around and braced myself as we waded into the convivial setting that flowed with alcohol and conversational questions such as, "What do you do for a living?" I felt reluctant to go into any details about my now-defunct advertising career, and I was ashamed I didn't have anything else to offer. I worried I might be putting myself in a situation that could unwittingly work against my newfound health. Although John and I used to attend many plays earlier in our marriage, it had been years since we mingled with theatre folks, whose lives naturally burst with drama, laughter, and emotion. I feared I might feel swallowed up and overwhelmed, incapable of conducting myself appropriately. John assured me we wouldn't stay long, and if I felt uncomfortable we would leave immediately.

"It's so nice to meet you, Martha. How did you like the show?" A beautiful ingénue, still in her stage makeup, shook my hand as we were introduced. Fortunately a lengthy critique would never be heard over the noise level in the bar, so my pat reply sufficed.

"Wonderful. Loved it. You were marvelous." I can do this, I thought to myself. They're just people like me and, besides, they've probably got their own sad story hiding inside their hearts just like I do.

I soon regained my social bearings, and before I knew it I found a seat at a large, round table with several new acquaintances, all of us appreciating each other's gift of gab. My conversations with people felt alive and real. I sensed a direct connection with them that made our interaction authentic and important. The invisible wall that for so long had separated me from everyone in my life vanished. I was experiencing life in a new, visceral way.

At one point I looked around the table, fascinated with what I observed, and even more amazed at what I felt. *Wow, Martha—can you believe you're sitting here in a bar, at a party with strangers, and actually enjoying yourself?* Only a few months before, this scenario could never have happened. I would not have had the energy to step outside my depression cave, and even if I had the energy, I would not have had the courage to face others in a public place—a bar, no less.

At the time I didn't connect this unique sensation to TMS, but I subsequently learned that in some people, neural stimulation can actually enhance mental cognition. During my depression—and probably for most of my life—my perception of living felt like I was watching a movie or a video, separated from the action. Now, everything suddenly looked, sounded, and felt much clearer—more real and alive. As I scanned the faces around the table, instead of viewing my life on a screen, I felt as if I were in a live performance on a stage interacting with real people in real time. Studies indicate that patients see the world with a new clarity after their depression has lifted. Colors appear brighter, objects become more vibrant and clearly defined, and patients' ability to associate ideas improves after neurological stimulation. I began to notice my own brain operating at a new level of acuity. Finally I had a positive, helpful side effect instead of medication's weight gain and constipation.

In the midst of the noisy party, a wave of heartfelt gratitude washed over me. It felt good to be with people again. It felt good to know I could keep up my end of a conversation. It felt especially good to look across the table and catch John's admiring eyes as he witnessed my rebirth into a life worth living.

He winked. I blinked.

16 | THE OTHER MARTHA

Martha, Martha, you are worried and distracted by many things; there is need of only one thing. Mary has chosen the better part, which will not be taken away from her.

— Luke 10:38–42

Sitting at Sunday Mass sandwiched between other Catholic girls popularly named Mary, this eight-year-old Martha always winced when the priest read the New Testament Gospel about Jesus' visit to Martha and Mary's house.

On said occasion, Martha slaved away in the kitchen preparing a special meal for their mystic friend, Jesus, who had just resurrected their brother Lazarus from the dead. Younger sister Mary adoringly plopped herself at the foot of the Master in the living room, captivated with his presence. When Martha got cranky and complained because Mary wasn't helping out with the food, Jesus chided her, told her to get over it, and instead pay attention to his pearls of wisdom.

By the end of Father O'Neill's holy reading, I always felt vicariously scolded. I imagined that all the girls to my left and right with the then popular name Mary beamed with self-satisfaction since their name, tacitly endorsed by the priest from the pulpit, put them on Jesus' A-Team. I invariably cringed as I shrunk into the hard, oak church pew fervently wishing my parents had come up with a less incriminating moniker for their third child.

Fast-forward ten years…

As much as I detested my name, I unconsciously lived up to Bible Martha's obsessive reputation in all things domestic. I enrolled in every available home economics class throughout junior high and high school—cooking in the fall semesters, sewing every spring. My most treasured high school graduation gift was the official Good Housekeeping Cookbook with many pages now marked by the butter, vanilla, and cinnamon stains bearing witness to the recipes I prepared.

My older sister, Maria, married during the summer I turned sixteen. It was one of those simple, homegrown weddings. As her maid of honor, a role I particularly cherished, I put myself in charge of cooking the prenuptial rehearsal dinner for her new in-laws. My mother, in her never-ending support for her children's ambitions, happily relinquished her kitchen to me. The groom's family drove in from eight hundred miles away the day before the ceremony. About the same time they wiped their North Carolinian chins with the wedding bell-embossed paper napkins, they showered me with endless praise for the spread I set out for everyone.

My sister's new mother-in-law declared, "Oh, Martha, I've never had such delicious beans—how long did you bake them with that maple syrup? And please send me that recipe for the Jewel Salad—it's so pretty and unique."

The Jewel Salad consisted of variously flavored Jell-O cubes creatively suspended in a whipped mousse mold. The grape-flavored gelatin produced deep purple garnets, strawberry became the rubies, orange the topaz, lime the emeralds, and lemon the ceremony-appropriate diamonds. Once turned out of the molded pan onto a chilled, decorative plate, the end result looked like a crown of brightly colored jewels. As my culinary horizons broadened and gained sophistication, I never again made another Jell-O mold—jeweled or otherwise. But creating the menu for my first big party at the age of sixteen and getting everything to turn out right took skills I felt proud to possess. This early success set me squarely on my "presentation is everything" course.

Before I graduated from high school, my father's oldest sister visited us from Pittsburgh. We hardly knew Aunt Anne since she lived so far away and wasn't much of a world traveler, but when she offered to make authentic Polish halupkies for our dinner one night, I became her shadow. I sponged up every step of the old family recipe filed away in her Ukrainian, gray-haired head. When she departed, I assumed the position of the official family stuffed cabbage cook from then on.

Fast-forward ten more years…

During my young-wife-and-mother years, holidays, birthdays, and even funeral gatherings bore my own "Martha" hospitality signature. I found comfort, satisfaction, and significance in everything from sewing a window treatment, to wrapping gifts with elaborate bows, to rolling out pie dough for a deep-dish apple pie. The red and blue ribbons garnered by the baked goods I entered in the Cannondale Grange Fair hung proudly in my kitchen for all to see. The year I finally won the coveted "Best in Show" purple ribbon delicately accented with white lace put a satisfying and final garnish on my quest for culinary recognition.

Fast-forward to my late fifties…

The days of planning menus, hosting parties, and maintaining my Martha-Wannabe-Stewart image disappeared when I descended into the abyss of major depression. As my advertising career evaporated, so did all aspirations to cook or sew, much less eat or maintain a household. The failed suicide attempt, two weeks in hospitals followed by ten months of unsuccessful medication treatment trials, and countless hours of psychotherapy had redefined my life. I lacked the energy to even shop for groceries, much less plan a menu or prepare a meal for John and me. Mentally, physically, and emotionally I detached myself from those years of daunting domesticity. It was the Other Martha who set that perfect table. The Other Martha who whipped up the comforting pot of soup for the friend in need or supplied the kids' nursery school with eighteen dozen cookies for the open house night. When I became ill with depression, the Other Martha disappeared with all the extra platters, plates, chafing dishes, tablecloths, and entertaining paraphernalia I willingly packed up and gave to my younger sister. It was someone else's turn to do the hosting and roasting for any gatherings.

By mid-August, after I completed the six weeks of TMS therapy, I noticed how I began to enjoy spending more time trolling the aisles of our local food market. The smells of the bakery teased my salivary glands for a slice of warm crusty bread. The summer's generous crops of fruits and vegetables beckoned to me through the hydrating mist softly settling on their vibrantly colored skins.

Hmmm. I bet those peaches would make a fabulous upside-down cake. Do I still have that cobbler pan? Maybe I could make a peach cobbler with blueberries for added color.

My reinvigorated senses were just another indication that TMS was working. The lift I felt from the magnetic pulses began pulling me out of the darkness. I felt recharged and ready to resume a healthy, productive life after the six weeks of daily treatments. Suddenly a trunk load of groceries followed me home from the grocery store, and my culinary juices flowed just about every night of the week after that. John never complained about the meager pickings he'd foraged during the previous year, but whenever I set a plate of homemade anything before him, his enthusiastic, "Honey, this is delicious. Thank you so much for making such a wonderful dinner," encouraged me to reopen my abandoned cookbooks.

∽◡∾

The summer I completed my TMS treatments drew to a close—and my blue mood right along with it—I felt grateful for the new energy and lightness. It also felt good not dragging through each day like a hopeless case. I surprised myself by organizing a long-overdue get-together with some treasured friends with whom I had lost touch during my isolation months.

I longed to reconnect, to be with women whose lives mattered to themselves and to the people around them. Their immediate and positive response to my phone calls assured me I hadn't lost their friendship.

We decided to hold our gathering at my friend Lisa's parents' home, since it was the most conveniently located place for everyone. I had been a frequent guest there since our college days in Boston, where we began our lifelong friendship. The elegant house commanded an expansive hill, comfortably overlooking Long Island Sound. Dining on the patio perched high above the sloping, landscaped yard that led down to the enticing swimming pool seemed the ideal spot for a perfect summertime ladies' luncheon.

The house itself held many special memories for me over the past thirty years. Holidays, birthdays, funerals, and weddings—all had taken place at this magnificent, spacious home. The sunken living room, with twin baby grand pianos, provided a natural stage for the many talented musicians, singers, and actors who regularly attended the always anticipated lavish affairs. My contribution for the festivities came out of the oven rather than the baby grand, and I never failed to earn rave reviews. Platters of handmade savory appetizers, steaming trays of lemony chicken paillards, and decadent desserts well worth every single calorie headlined my repertoire.

During the time I lived in the depression cave, my unusual absence at these parties had not gone unnoticed by our many friends. I'm sure Lisa's evasive and protective response to "Where's Martha?" left everyone in a quandary. The choices for me were troublesome: show up and chance failure at keeping up the everything-is-fine charade, or isolate myself in a shroud of secrecy and subject myself to a flurry of speculation. I defaulted to the latter with unmitigated cowardice.

Now that I felt happier over a year later, I decided to test my long-unused entertaining skills with a simple but elegant menu and a few friends who would understand if my experiment failed. Regardless, I knew in my heart that a bucket of KFC chicken would have been just fine with them.

Since I had initiated the get-together, I naturally offered to bring the meal, although the second the words escaped my lips I gulped with uncertainty that I could pull it off. Up until that moment, I honestly believed I would never be cooking for anyone ever again—and here I was offering to do the whole shebang.

"I'll be there by 12:30, Lisa. I'm bringing a nice lunch for us. Poached fresh salmon over wild rice salad with blanched haricots vert. Nothing fussy. Sweet melon and tart mango sorbet for dessert. Just make sure there's plenty of ice for the tea."

The unexpected satisfaction I experienced in creatively planning the fare, methodically shopping for the food, carefully preparing and proudly serving it, provided me a tremendous sense of relief from those self-doubts. As I set the four plates of poached salmon on the terrace table, worthy of any Food Channel's camera shot, I realized I had not lost my knack for delighting people with a delectable, beautifully presented meal. All three women reinforced my silent internal victory with their loud, effusive "oohs and aahs".

The luncheon itself could not have been easier to produce. The challenge remained in resurrecting my ability to intelligently participate in conversation, stay focused without becoming tearful, and settle comfortably into my own skin. My depression had robbed me of friendships for nearly two years. I hoped this re-entry into social interaction would be similar to the concept of "You never forget how to ride a bicycle."

Women have such a huge capacity to empathize with one another, especially women who have had their own mountains to climb, as certainly my three friends had over the many years we'd known each other. After lunch we bobbed around in the swimming pool in our Baby Boomer bodies for a while, chatting about the theatre and movies, good books, and traveling.

THE OTHER MARTHA

My friend Katherine was about to embark on a cross-country trip all by herself. She had recently returned from Florida, where she'd spent several months at her dying sister's side, whose passing sparked the "life is short" chord. So on her way back home to Connecticut, she bought a camper van and planned to retrace the scenic route John Steinbeck took when he wrote his legendary book, *Travels with Charlie.*

Another friend was grappling with the fact that her teenage son was about to go off to college. I'd already faced the empty nest dilemma. I was happy to impart any advice I derived from my own experience, which wasn't much, but at least I had something besides food to share.

No one pressed me about my troubles. No one needed to. I was obviously on the mend when I confidently delivered a tray of desserts to them as they sunned themselves poolside.

"Hooray, the old Martha's back!" Lisa triumphantly exclaimed as I deftly inserted a sprig of mint aside the fresh fruit and sorbet.

Before I could respond with a polite thank you, a surprising, instinctive reaction popped inside my head.

Wait a minute—I don't feel like the old Martha. I feel like a new and better Martha. And I honestly don't want to be the old Martha anymore.

Lisa's comment—and my unspoken gut reaction to it—stunned me with the truth that, although I clung to the life I mistakenly thought was so perfect before my illness, it no longer held any allure for me. Living my old days with depression while pretending everything was fine carried a burden I felt free to finally unload. My new days felt lighter, easier, and clearer now that I had found an effective, alternative way to deal with my illness. I didn't have to rely on medications and struggle with the side effects. The subtle, yet definite truce in my brain's battleground since I completed TMS allowed me to carry the day. I no longer felt afraid, uncertain, and inauthentic.

These three dear friends unknowingly sat as the beta site for the Reinvention of Martha. I smiled broadly, adjusted my apron, and asked, "Would anyone like more dessert?"

No one wondered more than I what the new Martha's world would look like. The only thing I knew for sure was that I was moving forward, convinced I should understand what happened to me, and more important, why—determined never to go back there again.

17 | TIME WILL TELL

"Time is the great physician."

– Benjamin Disraeli, *Endymion*

I opened the Christmas card without noticing the return address label stuck to the backside of the envelope. The greeting must have been overlooked during the flurry of activity that year, my second holiday season feeling happy, not depressed, and not medicated. The neatly handwritten message filled the entire left side of the card and spilled over atop the brightly printed sentiment, "It's a beautiful world and each of us is part of it. Season's Greetings!"

> Hi Martha—I think of you often and I remember being best friends. I saw you on the news a couple of weeks ago and couldn't believe my eyes— you are very brave and I applaud you for taking on the movement towards mental health—is that the way to say it? Listen, if you ever want to get together, even just the two of us, maybe we could meet in the middle for coffee or something.
>
> Love,
> Liz

Fortunately, voices from the past are sometimes able to break through even the staunchest barriers. During the months after my treatments, I began advocating for TMS public awareness including an interview Hartford Hospital asked me to do with a local television news station. Elizabeth, my very best friend from childhood in Hartford, had seen me on the broadcast.

I paused and thought about her comment for a moment. *But I did that news interview over a year ago.* I reexamined the envelope and in utter embarrassment I saw that the postage stamp was cancelled twelve months earlier. *This is a year-old Christmas card— and I'm just opening it now? How did it get past me last year, and how did it end up in this year's pile of cards?*

I immediately contacted Liz with an earnest apology for the oversight.

> January 21, 2012
> Dear Elizabeth,
>
> You must think me the most heartless, negligent person in the world! I was sifting through this year's Christmas cards to make sure I kept everyone's address and realized we had placed them in the same decorated bag with last year's cards (which I never sorted through, btw).
>
> I came across your card today, unopened, and have just now read it. I'm assuming it came last year since you've referenced the news interview I did around that same time for TMS. I can't begin to tell you how sorry I am that I never saw your message, but please know I am equally relieved that I at least discovered it now. In the meantime, I am so happy to hear from you and yes, we were best friends. My memories remain fond, clear, and cherished.
>
> Love,
> Martha

Within days of receiving my apology Elizabeth called me. In the twelve-plus months with no reply from me to her lovely holiday card, she said she assumed she had offended me with her allusion to mental health. Nothing could have been further from the truth. I felt relieved that the proverbial cat was out of the bag. I felt enormous gratitude that this painful experience incredibly led me to full disclosure and a reconnection with someone I held so dearly in my memories for over four decades.

~⁓

Two weeks later I arrived early at the restaurant where Elizabeth and I planned to rekindle our friendship. Since I was so belated in responding to her card, the last thing I wanted was to show up late for this long-overdue reunion. I waited in my car, pondering the nearly fifty years that kept us on separate life journeys when the Pasternack tribe had migrated to Florida from Connecticut in 1962. This unwelcomed relocation occurred when Elizabeth and I were inseparable and reaching our preteen, best-girlfriends-in-the-world stride—just at the point where the dolls and imaginary games no longer held their magic. We were ready to move on to the big-girl stuff our older sisters dangled before us—pop music, nylon stockings, lipstick, and boys. We never got to share notes about those things. I wondered if we'd have much more to talk about now.

At precisely twelve-thirty I checked my lipstick and hair in my car's rearview mirror and went into the restaurant. I worried if we'd even recognize each other now that time had laid claim to our complexion, hair, and girth. An energetic young man greeted me with an armful of large menus. I'm sure he could tell I was on a mission when I immediately started scoping out the place for the perfect table.

"Hi, I'm meeting an old friend for lunch and we haven't seen each other in years, so could we please have a quiet table in the corner," I asked as we glided through the dining room.

"Sure, but I got the same request from another lady I just seated. Is this your friend here?" He nodded to a booth against the wall as we approached it. No introductions needed—she looked the same, and I must not have changed all that much either because Elizabeth jumped up and warmly embraced me without hesitation. I nearly cried with relief and delight.

Time is such a trickster. It skews perceptions in the same way that looking through the opposite ends of a telescope does. Through one end, things look so close and real, but placing the other end to the eye pushes them so far away. I had the same feeling about seeing Elizabeth again.

As we hugged each other and settled into the cozy booth, I felt like the years between us mysteriously dissolved, but at the same moment—considering all we had missed out on in each other's lives—I worried we might feel like strangers. Thankfully, we didn't.

Neither of us knew where to begin our conversation. But the serendipitous TMS television interview, along with the unopened Christmas card, cracked open the shell holding the personal histories we both willingly shared over soup and salad. We reminisced about the old Hartford neighborhood and its array of long-gone Italian and Irish families. We gave updates about our siblings and mourned our deceased parents, adding footnotes about the accompanying emotional fallout, both positive and negative.

As I finally found the nerve to share the truth about my suicide attempt, I felt unexpectedly at ease about it. Recounting my collapse and recovery didn't require as much mental and emotional fortitude as it had in the past when I spoke of it to others. I realized how far I had come over the previous two and a half years—that I had reclaimed my life in a productive and satisfying way.

"It's shocking to know that I almost ended my life," I admitted. "I still can't believe I actually went so far down that dark path."

I couldn't detect even a shred of shock or disapproval in her eyes. She didn't ask me why I did it, or how my family reacted, or even if I was sorry. She simply accepted my story as a scrap of fabric in my life's multicolored quilt.

"Well, we've each had our personal journeys, and it's not for either of us or anyone else to judge, is it?" she said softly.

Her wisdom silenced me for a moment. I couldn't respond. She slowly stirred her tea, respecting the pause in our conversation. I let out a simple sigh. I needed a little open space to fully absorb the preciousness of the moment. I stared at the window on the far side of the room. The noonday sun had disappeared, and I sensed the late afternoon shadows signaling it was time to leave. Once again, time played its trick on me when I realized four and a half hours had slipped by in what seemed like only one.

We said goodbye in the parking lot with the promise we'd stay close. I'd already offered to help out with some details for her daughter's upcoming wedding as a subconscious guarantee we'd meet again.

During my drive home I thought to myself, I have come full circle. We have come full circle. Two best friends who have lived their entire lives apart, but who still share a special affection, a unique understanding. How absolutely remarkable.

The interesting thing about the concept of coming full circle is that although it insinuates an ending, in reality, a circle is endless. It goes round and round just as life revolves around each year's passing seasons. I now appreciate that coming full circle at this point in my life isn't an ending. The chapter with the dark story is just another phase that miraculously carried me to the start of another round of living.

How my marriage survived is another miracle.

Throughout the many months prior to receiving TMS, I became so detached from John he seemed almost invisible to me. We didn't have many conversations because he didn't know what to say or do, and in truth, I remained inconsolable. He constantly worried about what he'd find when he got home from school each day—whether I'd still be in bed, or if I was up, would I be agitated or in a misery pit. He stopped asking, "How are you today?" because he already knew the answer—I wanted to die—a truth too painful to hear.

But he still came home. And he stayed.

It wasn't a Hallmark-card-storybook-love-nest either. The dark days dragged on with each of us marooned on our separate islands—confused, frustrated and frightened.

It's not uncommon that a person will seek out a comfort zone when faced with a difficult situation, especially when it involves intense emotions. He or she will dive into an outside activity to escape strife at home. John didn't. He hung in there and went shoulder to shoulder with me as we muddled through what felt like a maze in an amusement park's House of Mirrors. He limited his time away from home so I wouldn't be left alone. He gave up his extra curricular activities such as a big band group he played in every week. He kept the household afloat, did the laundry and survived on a steady diet of pasta and quick-fix, frozen dinners.

When we talked about it after I began to feel well again, he simply said, "I felt like I was always walking on eggshells. I just didn't know what to do, so I kept quiet." But internally, he anguished over our future. He said he knew enough not to react to anything I said or did because any ingratiating sympathy or attempt to reason, cajole, or object would only have made matters worse.

John did the most heroic thing I believe anyone could do for another human being: he stayed present with his love for me. He didn't try to fix me, heal me, or reason with me. I never felt judged by him, nor did I feel pressured to "snap out of it" as most people assume a depressed person is capable of doing, which they are not.

I know how painful this has been for John, and I continue to feel regret for what he has had to endure on my account. But I know we have both come to a better understanding of depression as a bona fide illness.

John vigilantly guards our lifestyle to ensure I avoid the pitfalls of the disease. There are times when he notices my mood dipping before I do, and he encourages me to go for a maintenance TMS session. His constancy, understanding and unconditional love sustain me above all else.

∿

My life in advertising has ended, and I continue to grieve the loss of that career. Whenever I go into New York or meet up with my old marketing pals, I become wistful and a bit melancholy. But I'm putting that business experience to good use. I'm relying on the skills that got me into those corner offices for a more important mission—helping other patients with diagnosed depression navigate the health care and insurance systems.

I coach patients with depression, over the phone and in person, to give them my own patient experience with TMS and help them understand what it's all about. I assist them with their insurance appeal letters and we are now realizing increasing success with the insurance companies. In fact, at this printing, the insurance company in Connecticut that I challenged has just announced it will now be covering TMS therapy which means that patients will no longer have to go through the arduous appeal process I faced.

I've been blessed with meeting Dr. Randy Pardell thanks to a mutual friend whose name, ironically, is Joy. Together Dr. Pardell and I have begun monthly TMS support groups for patients who are either considering TMS, are currently in TMS therapy, or who have completed it.

These activities support my own psyche in ways I didn't anticipate. By focusing my attention toward someone else's concerns, I enjoy a sense of purpose. When I'm doing something good for someone else I always feel better. In fact, studies have proved that altruism—even the simplest act of kindness—induces a chemical reaction in the brain that promotes happiness. It's a positive feedback loop. The happier I feel, the more I am able to help others. It's my "Do good to feel good," strategy.

I also feel valued when Dr. Pardell and I do TMS medical education presentations for other doctors and clinicians who are now learning about this unique and effective psychiatric therapy. There is a pressing need to share our patient and physician TMS experience to help update their existing therapy toolkit. This enables them to offer information about every available alternative to their patients.

My life is full again. I have a compassionate therapist, a competent psychiatrist, and loving family and friends to thank for it. Moving forward with TMS as my go-to treatment for depression, the biggest hurdle I now face, post-TMS, is accepting depression as a chronic, physical, brain illness that directly affects my spirit. I know there is no medication or alternative therapy that will ever be able to deliver the keys to a life worth living. It's up to me to create a lifestyle that supports my recovery and manages my condition. And that challenge faces every person who suffers with clinical depression, whether they're treated by medications or by TMS therapy—or even ECT.

This is especially crucial when I recall how dark and hopeless I felt, and how easy it was to come to the decision to end my life. I consider depression my enemy and I'm on a constant lookout for its impact on my thoughts and feelings that nearly defeated me.

I know that my prospects for a happy future depend on my commitment to a determined spirit, self-discipline, courage, and truthfulness. There can be no more game face cover-ups where I pretend to everyone—including myself—that I'm fine when I'm not. On the other hand, I have to make sure I am, indeed, fine. I have to do my part to stay healthy and guard against a relapse. I'm fortunate to have an ongoing relationship with my talk therapist, Susan, whom I see whenever I sense a dark cloud forming. I'm equally fortunate that TMS has given my brain enough of a boost that I don't have to take antidepressant medications. My TMS maintenance plan is minimal—I'll periodically go for a single treatment that provides an adequate lift.

Since depression is an illusive and complicated illness that's rooted in the body (my brain) but presents itself in behavior (my mood and emotions), it's important for me to attend to both sides of the equation. This means avoiding people, places, and things that undermine my mental and emotional wellbeing. It also means I have to take care of myself—body and spirit.

To that end, I follow these simple, but important, guidelines.

• I do not consume alcohol. It is a depressant and will totally undermine everything else on this list if I break this rule.

• I eat nutritious meals that include a balance of protein, complex carbohydrates, fruits, and vegetables, and I try to avoid fat. I'm still working on staving off my sweet-tooth habit.

• Every day I take a multivitamin and Omega-3 and Vitamin D supplements.

• I get a good night's sleep, usually seven to eight hours. Before I doze off I consciously choose something positive and uplifting to ponder. Otherwise, I might slip into a negative rumination cycle that will prevent me from falling asleep easily.

• I walk my little Josie dog every day because exercise increases the activity of important brain chemicals such as dopamine and serotonin. (Full disclosure: Josie and I confess we should exercise more.)

• I make a conscious effort to engage in interpersonal activities. I offer to help friends. I show up for family events and schedule dates with former colleagues. I've attended a few writers' conferences and I'm in a weekly writers group that offers me support not only for my writing, but personally as well.

Interacting with others also provides me with subtle feedback as to how well I'm doing. For example, whenever someone paid me a compliment in the past, an inner voice would always refute it with "God, if you only knew how ugly I feel inside you'd never say that." Now social gatherings are much more fun because I'm able to respond to "Hey, Martha, you're looking great!" with a genuine "Thank you!"—without feeling like a fraud wearing a happy-face mask.

On the other hand, since I've gone public with my illness and my family and friends are tuned into my situation, I'm confident they'll let me know if I appear to be drifting toward the dark side.

• I avoid unnecessary stressful situations like over scheduling my days or going to places that are too noisy, crowded, or physically and/or emotionally demanding. I also notice that if there's not enough time to get something accomplished, I'll reschedule it or eliminate it from my "To Do List", because working with unrealistic deadlines is a stressor. If one sneaks up on me, however, I quickly and mindfully take a deep breath and step away from it, because I know that undue stress will set off a negative chemical reaction for a healthy brain.

• I try to stay conscious of people who are overly negative and unsupportive of me and of others. I'm thankful to have a wealth of uplifting friends and family, so this isn't a huge issue. But there can be times in life when a toxic person shows up unannounced. It's important for me to be on the lookout for anyone whom I feel picks away at my spirit and keep him or her at an arm's length.

• I take a moment to think before I say "Yes" to someone's request and allow myself to say "No" if I feel I'll be inflicting a negative situation upon myself—and ultimately on them—when I realize I should never have agreed to it and succumb to the subsequent pressure. Following my intuition and saying "No" to something I really don't want to do (but used to agree to out of guilt) is actually saying "Yes" to my mental healthfulness.

• Usually before I go to bed, I write a list for the next day so I know what I'm expecting of myself. Its physical existence gets me out of bed in the morning. Also, setting realistic goals and achieving them supports my self-esteem and assures me that I'm fully engaged in life. It feels gratifying to cross out items on the list, and at the end of the day I have proof that I got something done.

And even though I don't always get everything accomplished, at least I know I'm making a gallant effort. Whatever's left over I either move to the next day's list or decide it wasn't that important in the first place.

• Last, I try to meditate almost every day for at least thirty to forty-five minutes. Meditation has enabled me to become more mindful, more creative, calmer, and more connected to my inner voice—the one that guides me to insights and a peaceful perspective about life. Sometimes I just sit quietly and do conscious, simple breathing using Dr. Andrew Weil's and Dr. Jon Kabat-Zinn's techniques. Other times I use guided meditation CDs that talk me through meditative exercises and visualizations. I finish my meditations with a few simple affirmations such as "Every day in every way I'm getting better and better." Or one of my favorites, "Miracles are happening in my life here and now."

Miracles *are* happening in my life here and now—because you are reading this book. My wish for you is that you'll discover a glimmer of hope in your heart and be able to welcome miracles into your own life.

FREQUENTLY ASKED QUESTIONS

By Randy Ian Pardell, MD DFAPA

I am fortunate to have been in psychiatric practice during an era of great advances and breakthroughs in treatments of psychiatric disorders. In 1984, at the start of my psychiatry residency training at St. Luke's-Roosevelt Hospital in New York City, medicines such as Thorazine, Elavil, and Lithium were used to control psychiatric conditions, albeit with many unwanted side effects. As a physician, the lack of effective and tolerable medication options for my patients was frustrating.

I sought out a research elective at Columbia University College of Physicians and Surgeons with Alexander Glassman MD, Director of the Department of Clinical Psychopharmacology. At the time, Dr. Glassman was the world's preeminent expert on antidepressant medication and pioneered the study on evaluation of antidepressant medication blood levels to determine therapeutic effectiveness. I recall a conversation we had in early 1987 when I asked, "Are the current antidepressant medications actually effective?" to which he responded, "Depression is a physiological disorder like any other medical illness. Antidepressants work, but we need medications that work better and are well-tolerated." During my time at Columbia, I was exposed to groundbreaking research that would become future treatment modalities in psychiatry.

In December of 1987, as Chief Resident in Psychiatry, I had my first chance to prescribe Prozac, which was the greatest advancement in psychiatry in more than twenty-five years. My patient was an acutely ill woman suffering from severe depression and suicidality, and who had been treated with many of the available antidepressant medications but could not tolerate any of them. Finally a medication existed that was effective for her with side effects that were more easily borne.

The advent of Prozac and other SSRI antidepressants lead the way for the acceptance of psychiatric medications for the general population. These compounds did not have the severe cardiac side effects, dry mouth, constipation, or weight gain associated with tricyclic antidepressants. When my wife and I moved to the Mid Hudson Valley of New York in the late 1980's, Prozac had become a household word. As the "Decade of the Brain" unfolded in the 1990s, multiple new SSRI and SNRI antidepressants followed as research expanded and treatment options increased. My medication arsenal included Zoloft, Paxil, and Effexor, which yielded positive patient outcomes, but over time patients began to complain about sexual side effects, weight gain, and withdrawal effects.

In the early and mid-1990s atypical antipsychotics such as Risperdal and Zyprexa were developed. These revolutionary medications treated Schizophrenia and Bipolar Disorder without the movement problems or cognitive dulling of conventional antipsychotics. Yet patients were still experiencing significant side effects—like weight gain coupled with elevations of undesirable cholesterol and lipids—predisposing them to diabetes and heart disease.

Into the 2000s research advances continued with new compounds released that attempted to minimize the burden of side effects. However, I still struggled with the patients who did not respond to the available medications or who could not tolerate their side effects. There was still a missing treatment option that needed to be uncovered.

In 2006, well entrenched in my private practice of general psychiatry and psychopharmacology, a long-standing patient challenged me to find an effective treatment for his depression that did not cause him the side effects of cognitive dulling and fatigue. Alternative treatment options meant Electroconvulsive Treatment (ECT), an option he summarily declined when I described the possible side effects of ECT and potential for long-term memory impairment.

Looming on the horizon, however, was a new treatment option—Transcranial Magnetic Stimulation (TMS). Although the science of TMS had been around for almost twenty years, its application to neuroscience and psychiatry was finally being clinically tested. TMS employs the familiar magnetic pulse used in MRI technology to treat depression by targeting areas of the brain responsible for depression. A clinical trial of the Neurostar TMS Therapy® system was taking place at Columbia University. I connected with the lead investigator, Sarah Lisanby MD, and suggested my patient for the clinical trial.

In October 2008 the Neurostar TMS Therapy® was FDA approved, and soon after my patient wanted to know when I would be offering TMS treatment in my practice. Intrigued, I contacted Neuronetics, the developer of the Neurostar TMS Therapy system, for information.

Shortly after my inquiry, Neuronetics invited me to Philadelphia for their Pioneer's Meeting, a gathering of the first psychiatrists in the country who were treating patients with TMS therapy. It was an illuminating conference. A palpable air of excitement filled the room as one doctor after another discussed the positive outcomes of this innovative technology. One of the world's leading TMS experts, Mark George MD, lectured on his fifteen years of TMS research. He showed PET scans of a patient's brain after receiving TMS treatment and contrasted them with the scans taken before treatment. TMS stimulated the brain causing a normalization of blood flow and brain activity thus abating the depression, yet without the side effects associated with antidepressant medication. A remarkable display of quantified data convinced me of the undeniable benefits of this treatment.

We opened the doors of the TMS Center of the Hudson Valley in December 2009, and have treated more than sixty patients to date. Our second center in Saratoga Springs, NY opened in January 2012. The ability to transform my patients' lives has been the most satisfying experience of my psychiatric career. I continue to lecture around the country about TMS and have interested other psychiatrists, mental health clinicians, and patients about the potential of TMS to treat psychiatric conditions.

Martha Rhodes and I have begun one of the first TMS support groups in the nation and have listened to patients as they recall their frustration with medication therapy, lack of awareness about TMS by psychiatrists, and satisfaction when TMS helped them recover when medications did not.

Over the past three years, I have seen TMS therapy grow in awareness as a treatment for severe depression, but there is much more to do. My hope is that *3,000 Pulses* and Martha's story will drive potential patients and mental health clinicians to learn more about this "transformational" treatment and move TMS to general clinical and insurance acceptance.

The following information should answer any questions you may have about TMS. They are the same questions asked by almost every patient I've treated either before or during their TMS therapy.

Randy Ian Pardell, MD DFAPA
July 2012

What is depression?

Depressive disorders are medical illnesses that afflict up to nineteen million U.S. citizens a year, and over their lifetime nearly 17% of our population will suffer from its most severe form— Major Depressive Disorder (depression). Depression is twice as common in women as it is in men. Two percent of our population suffers from severe depression that disables people from being able to work and engage in normal social functioning.

All of us will have feelings of sadness, but most of the time these feelings pass quickly within a few hours or days. Depression is a profound illness—with both emotional and physical symptoms—that lasts more than two weeks and, typically, for months and years. The emotional symptoms include persistent sadness, anxiety, and "empty" feelings. There is a loss of interest or pleasure in the activities that normally bring pleasure. There are feelings of hopelessness, helplessness, and negativity. People feel worthless, down on themselves, and guilt-ridden. Those afflicted experience irritability and difficulty in concentrating and in making decisions.

Many patients with depression suffer from suicidal thinking and behavior as a means of escaping the emotional pain associated with the disorder. Suicide is the eighth leading cause of death in the United States and the third leading cause of death in young adults age fifteen to twenty-four, with two-thirds of suicide victims suffering from depression.

The physical symptoms of depression include insomnia and early morning awakening with an inability to get back to sleep, although a minor proportion of patients sleep excessively. People with depression lose their appetite and often lose more than 5% of their body weight when depressed. Conversely, another portion of patients may eat more and gain weight during depression. People suffering with depression are restless and agitated; they experience fatigue and a profound slowing down of energy level. Others can experience aches, pains, headaches, and gastrointestinal problems such as constipation, diarrhea, nausea, and indigestion.

What causes depression?

Major Depressive Disorder is caused by the interaction between genes and environment along with biological and psychological factors. It is a brain disease that is associated with disorders of neurotransmitters, which are the chemicals that nerve cells use to communicate, and abnormal information processing of brain circuits. There are hormonal changes in depression as stress hormones are out of balance, and the structure of the brain changes with depression as seen on MRI scans of the brain with shrinking of important brain regions.

Some types of depression run in families and scientists have isolated certain genes that predispose people toward depression. Major life events such as the loss of a loved one or emotionally traumatic experiences can trigger depressive episodes.

Depression can last for months or years if left untreated although with medication therapy, lifestyle changes, and psychotherapy, many depression sufferers can return to normal mood and functioning. However, only 30% of patients with a standard antidepressant medication treatment get well. Even after extensive medication trials and psychotherapy, nearly one-third of depression sufferers remain symptomatic. Given these results, there is a strong need for alternative treatments for Major Depressive Disorder such as the Transcranial Magnetic Stimulation (TMS) described in this book.

What is TMS therapy?

TMS stands for Transcranial Magnetic Stimulation. Transcranial indicates that magnetic energy crosses through the cranial (head) bone and into the brain itself. Magnetic means that magnetic energy is sent to the area that clinicians want to stimulate. Magnetism has been described for centuries, dating back even earlier than ancient Greece. Aristotle wrote a scientific treatise on magnetism in the fourth century BC. A century earlier, the first reported medical use of magnets was by an Indian surgeon named Sushruta. But it wasn't until 1831 that British physicist Michael Faraday formulated the connection between electricity and magnetism when he determined that a time-varying magnetic field induces electric currents in conductive surfaces. Faraday's law of electromagnetism is the basis of modern-day TMS treatment.

The first solid-state TMS machine used for medical purposes was invented by Anthony Barker, MD, in Sheffield, England, in 1985. He was looking for a way to map brain areas in patients affected by stroke. Electricity was not practical for this purpose, as the cranium (skull bone) does not conduct electricity well. Dr. Barker realized that when you have a hard, non-conductive surface, magnetic energy goes through easily. (Remember as a child playing with magnets? You could move metal on top of a table by directing the magnet under the table top.) During the time that Dr. Barker was brain mapping stroke victims with TMS, a curious finding occurred. Patients began to feel better and less depressed. This finding promoted research in using TMS (rTMS, repetitive transcranial magnetic stimulation over days and weeks) to treat a variety of neuropsychiatric conditions including Major Depressive Disorder.

TMS therapy is used to treat depression by stimulating the brain non-invasively using an electromagnetic field, similar to those magnetic fields produced by an MRI machine. During TMS therapy, a magnetic field is administered in very short pulses to the part of the brain (the dorsolateral prefrontal cortex which is the front left part of the brain) that research has demonstrated is associated with depression. The typical initial course of treatment is about thirty-seven minutes daily over four to six weeks.

How does TMS therapy work?

TMS therapy uses short pulses of magnetic fields to stimulate the prefrontal cortex of the brain which is thought to function differently in patients with depression. The prefrontal cortex is located in the front part of the brain and is responsible for executive functions such as problem solving, cognitive and motor planning, verbal working memory, and mental energy. This area of the brain is connected to deeper structures in the brain associated with emotional functioning, including the areas that control the depressive symptoms of anxiety, sad mood, and sleep and appetite dysfunctions occurring with clinical depression.

The human brain has more than 100 billion nerve cells with up to 15,000 connections for each nerve cell. There are more connections in our brains than there are stars in the observed universe. The brain is an extensive electrochemical highway system that processes information. The magnetic fields from TMS produce an electric current in the brain that stimulates nerve cells (neurons) both electrically and chemically. This process awakens circuits in the brain that are underperforming and underfunctioning, and it creates new patterns for healthy connections. There is also release of neurotransmitters such as dopamine, serotonin, and norepinephrine, which are the same neurochemicals affected by antidepressant medication.

MRI scans of those afflicted with depression show that certain circuits begin to shrink over time. For instance, the hippocampus part of the brain that is responsible for semantic memory (long-term cognitive knowledge) and emotional control contracts in size under the influence of depression. The prefrontal cortex (the area we stimulate with TMS) also shows reduced activity on functional brain scans (PET/SPECT/fMRI) in depression. The process of TMS therapy stimulates the formation of peptides in nerve cells, such as BDNF (brain-derived neurotrophic factor), which act like a brain fertilizer. These substances cause nerve cells to branch out and connect, resulting in changes in the brain that are thought to be beneficial in the treatment of depression. TMS treatment restores function and structure to the areas that have been affected by depression.

Is TMS therapy a good alternative for patients who cannot tolerate the side effects associated with antidepressant medications?

Most of the common antidepressants produce unwanted side effects such as weight gain, loss of sexual interest, emotional numbing, sedation, and gastrointestinal symptoms. TMS is non-systemic (it does not circulate in the blood or throughout the body), so it does not have side effects associated with antidepressant medication. The most common side effects reported with TMS during clinical trials were headache and/or scalp pain or discomfort—generally mild to moderate—occurring less frequently after the first week of treatment. Less than 5% of patients in the NeuroStar TMS Therapy® clinical trials stopped due to adverse events.

Neurostar TMS Therapy® was approved by the U.S. Food and Drug Administration (FDA) in October 2008 for the treatment of patients with depression who have failed to achieve satisfactory improvement from one prior antidepressant medication at adequate dose and duration but who still did not get better. TMS therapy may not work for all patients with depression. In the Neurostar® clinical trials over half of patients responded to TMS therapy and nearly one-third were completely well by the end of the six-week clinical trial. In practices throughout the country similar effectiveness of TMS has been shown. You should speak with your doctor to determine if TMS therapy is an appropriate treatment option for you.

Is TMS therapy like other alternative therapies that use magnets to treat some illnesses?

No. TMS therapy involves a unique method of using pulsed magnetic fields for therapeutic benefit. The intensity of the magnetic field is similar to that of the magnetic fields used in magnetic resonance imaging, or MRI. These techniques differ radically from the use of low intensity, static magnetic fields. These products deliver weak and undirected static fields that are not capable of activating brain cells or treating a serious condition such as depression.

Is TMS therapy similar to Electroconvulsive Therapy (ECT)?

No, the two procedures are very different. Although both treatments stimulate the brain and are effective in the treatment of depression, there are many differences in safety and tolerability.

During the TMS therapy procedure, a magnetic pulse is administered to the front left part of the head which converts into a gentle electrical stimulation that awakens the part of the brain that is underfunctioning. Patients sit comfortably in a chair and are awake and alert throughout the entire thirty-seven-minute procedure—no sedation or anesthesia is used with TMS therapy. Patients can transport themselves to and from treatment.

Electroconvulsive Therapy (ECT)—or "Shock Therapy"— intentionally causes a seizure. ECT has been used around the world for more than seventy years to treat severe depression, catatonia, and manic psychosis. It is an effective treatment for these conditions; however, patients receiving ECT must be sedated with general anesthesia and paralyzed with muscle relaxants in an operating room setting in a hospital with anesthesia support and EEG and EKG monitoring.

With ECT an electrical charge is administered either to one side (unilateral) or both sides (bilateral) of the head and a seizure is induced. A seizure is a storm of electrical activity that surges throughout the brain and can last between thirty to sixty seconds. The reason why anesthesia is provided is to prevent involuntary movements that would result in a non-anaesthetized person. The seizure is believed to release neurotransmitters and neurotrophic factors that aid in the treatment of depression and other conditions.

FREQUENTLY ASKED QUESTIONS

A typical treatment course of ECT is three times a week for a total of eight to twelve treatments and sometimes more. Recovery from an ECT treatment session occurs slowly in a hospital recovery room, and patients are usually closely monitored for minutes or hours after a treatment. Patients are required to have a family member or friend drive them home from the ECT treatment, as post-ECT confusion can last for a few hours.

Short-term confusion and memory loss are common with ECT, and long-term disruptions in memory have been shown to occur and may persist indefinitely in some people. Because of the side effects associated with ECT, a significant amount of caregiver support is required during the treatment course.

In over 10,000 active treatments with Neurostar® TMS Therapy in clinical trials, no seizures were observed. TMS therapy was also shown to have no negative effects on memory function in clinical studies. However, there is a remote risk of seizure with TMS therapy. In the post-marketing NeuroStar TMS Therapy® surveillance, a low incidence of seizures has been reported. Some of these seizures were associated with the use of TMS in patients who were on medications that raised seizure risk or in which the TMS magnetic coil was placed in an incorrect location. The incidence of seizure is approximately 0.003% per treatment, and the incidence per treatment course is less than 0.1%.

Antidepressant medications have been associated with seizure risk according to their package inserts. TMS has a rare risk of seizure that is 0.1% per acute treatment course.

What is a typical course of treatment with TMS therapy?

In the Neurostar TMS Therapy® clinical trials, patients received TMS therapy five times per week for thirty-seven-minute sessions over four to six weeks. Some patients may respond sooner and others may require longer treatment. Patients treated with TMS therapy should receive treatment for a minimum of four weeks with additional treatments based on clinical judgment.

Who can provide TMS therapy?

Neurostar TMS Therapy® can only be provided by a licensed psychiatrist who has completed extensive education by Neuronetics training staff.

There are over 400 TMS centers around the continental United States and Hawaii. Three-quarters of Neurostar TMS centers are owned by private psychiatrists providing TMS in their local communities while the remaining quarter are operated within medical or academic centers. You can locate a nearby Neurostar TMS provider through Neuronetics' "Doctor Locator" on their website: www.neurostar.com.

Are there any side effects with TMS therapy?

Throughout over 10,000 active treatments performed in clinical trials, the most commonly reported side effects related to treatment were scalp discomfort and/or headache during treatment sessions. These side effects were generally mild to moderate and occurred less frequently after the first week of treatment. Less than 5% of patients treated with this TMS therapy discontinued treatment due to side effects.

These side effects (local site sensitivity and/or headache) occur in a third to half of patients. The psychiatrist or TMS clinician has the ability to adjust the strength of TMS stimulation to gradually acclimate each patient to the TMS treatment. Also the angle and position of the magnetic coil can be adjusted so that any uncomfortable stimulation of superficial nerves can be avoided which allows TMS therapy to be universally well-tolerated.

NeuroStar TMS therapy delivers a magnetic field that could cause metal objects that are within twelve inches from the device to move or get hot. NeuroStar TMS therapy is contraindicated in patients with implanted metallic devices or non-removable metallic objects in or around the head. Dental amalgam fillings are not affected by TMS.

**Do I need to have someone drive me to and from
TMS Therapy?**

For the first session of motor threshold determination, most patients should come with a family member, caregiver, or friend who can drive him or her home. Most patients are excited to start TMS and the anxiety associated with initiating a new treatment may make someone fatigued after their first TMS treatment. However, most patients can drive or walk to their subsequent TMS sessions without difficulty.

How long does it take to get results from TMS therapy?

Most patients will start to see improvement in depression symptoms by the fourth week. Some may respond sooner and others later. The earliest we have seen patients showing response was within the second week, while others may experience worsening of their depression before they begin to see improvement of their symptoms. Some patients may show improvement in energy soon after their treatment begins. For most patients, the robust response usually begins between the third and fourth weeks. A smaller number of patients will require more than thirty sessions to show improvement.

What is the success rate for TMS?

In the NeuroStar TMS Therapy® clinical trials, the success rate was over 50% of patients responded with a 50% reduction in symptoms on the Hamilton Depression Rating Scale with TMS alone and without antidepressant medication; 33% of patients went into full remission of their depressive symptoms. A recent NeuroStar TMS Therapy® Treatment Outcomes and Utilization Study, which evaluated over 300 patients treated at TMS centers across the country, reported that nearly 60% of patients responded with TMS treatment.

How many patients have undergone the treatment and what percentage of patients got relief from depression with TMS?

As of March 2012 over 8,500 patients have been treated with the Neurostar TMS Therapy® with nearly 250,000 treatments given across the United States. There are nearly 400 TMS centers in the country and the number is expanding as more patients are getting treated by—and responding to—TMS.

What are the potential risks of TMS therapy?

Neurostar TMS Therapy® is well tolerated and has been proven to be safe in clinical trials. In the Neurostar® clinical trials, over 10,000 TMS treatments demonstrated its safety, with no occurrence of seizures. However, there is a small risk of a seizure occurring during treatment.

Although TMS therapy has been proven effective, not all patients will benefit from it. Patients should be carefully monitored for worsening symptoms, signs or symptoms of suicidal behavior, and/or unusual behavior. Families and caregivers should also be aware of the need to observe patients and notify their treatment provider if symptoms worsen.

Who should not receive TMS therapy?

TMS therapy should not be used (is contraindicated) in patients with implanted metallic devices or non-removable metallic objects in or around the head. TMS therapy should be used with caution in patients with implanted devices that are controlled by physiological signals. This includes pacemakers and implantable cardioverter defibrillators (ICDs). It should be used in caution with patients using wearable cardioverter defibrillators.

Does TMS therapy cause brain tumors?

No. TMS therapy uses the same type and strength of magnetic fields as MRIs (magnetic resonance imaging), which have been used in tens of millions of patients around the world and have not been shown to cause tumors. The magnetic energy used in a full course of TMS therapy is less than what is received from one brain scan with an MRI. Over the past thirty years of brain MRI scanning, this technique has been shown to be safe without increased incidence of brain tumors or other central nervous system illness.

Does TMS therapy cause memory loss?

No. TMS therapy was systematically evaluated for its effects on memory. Clinical trials demonstrated that Neurostar® TMS therapy does not result in any negative effects on memory or concentration.

Is TMS therapy uncomfortable? What TMS therapy does feel like? Does it hurt?

The most common side effect related to treatment is scalp pain or discomfort during treatment sessions—which was described as mild to moderate. Some of our patients have termed the TMS treatment sensation as feeling "tapped by a woodpecker."

If necessary, you can treat this discomfort with an over-the-counter analgesic. If these side effects persist, your doctor can temporarily reduce the strength of the magnetic field pulses being administered or change the angle or position of the coil in order to make treatment more comfortable. Almost all patients will tolerate TMS and complete a full course of treatment.

How long does the antidepressant effect last?
Will I need any therapy beyond the first four to six weeks?
What happens after I complete TMS therapy?
Is TMS maintenance required and, if so, what is a usual maintenance program?

Depression is a highly recurrent illness for most patients and may require ongoing treatment. After completing the initial TMS therapy, patients may receive additional TMS treatment ordered by their psychiatrist if symptoms return. Frequency and number of treatments are determined by the clinical judgement of the psychiatrist.

In the original Neurostar TMS Therapy® clinical trials, all patients who responded to TMS therapy were transitioned to an antidepressant medication. They were then followed for six months. If patients fell back into depression, additional sessions were allowed. "Booster" TMS treatment was required by 37% of patients, and 85% of these patients returned to full remission of their depression symptoms; 63% did not require any additional TMS treatments and continued to feel well. In total nearly 90% of patients at the end of six months maintained their positive response.

Can I also take antidepressant(s) if I am receiving TMS therapy?

Yes. In clinical trials, Neurostar® TMS therapy was safely administered with and without other antidepressant medications. There is no contraindication for the combined use of TMS and antidepressant medication. However, if patients are changing doses of medication during the TMS treatment, it might be necessary for the psychiatrist to perform another motor threshold to determine if the treatment parameters have changed after starting or stopping a medication.

Does FDA clearance of the TMS therapy system mean that all TMS devices can be used to treat major depression within the United States?

No. The NeuroStar TMS Therapy® system is the first and only TMS device to be approved by the U.S. Food and Drug Administration (FDA) for the treatment of major depression. The TMS therapy system is also the first TMS device to have been evaluated and found effective in a large, multicenter, controlled clinical trial for the treatment of depression.

No other TMS device can claim to be FDA-cleared for the treatment of depression. There are a number of companies who are manufacturing other TMS devices. Brainsway® developed a "Deep TMS" device and Magventure® manufactures the Magpro System® Both are being tested in the U.S. in multicenter clinical trials for treatment of depression. It may be a number of years before these systems are cleared by the FDA and actively used clinically.

Does TMS therapy work in disorders besides depression?

NeuroStar TMS Therapy® has only systematically been evaluated in patients with unipolar, non-psychotic major depression. While there is promising data utilizing other TMS devices in a variety of additional neuropsychiatric disorders, these data are preliminary and require systematic evaluation in controlled clinical trials.

Clinical trials are underway for expanded use of TMS. Research utilizing TMS therapy is evolving in stroke rehabilitation, Traumatic Brain Injury (TBI), Parkinson's Disease, Alzheimer's Disease, chronic pain, Post Traumatic Stress Disorder, Bipolar Depression, Generalized Anxiety Disorder, Attention Deficit Hyperactivity Disorder and Migraine Headaches. You can find out more about the TMS clinical trials for a variety of disorders on http//:clinicaltrials.gov. These are closely controlled, scientific research studies involving patients and volunteers. Once the trials are completed, detailed analysis of the data will result in published findings about the efficacy of the TMS treatment for the disorder being studied.

Will TMS therapy be covered by my insurance and/or Medicare?

Whenever there is a new technology, insurers are often slow to adopt the new treatment until a significant number of patients have been treated and the treatment has been studied with scientific rigor. NeuroStar TMS Therapy® has been evaluated thoroughly in two randomized placebo-controlled clinical trials which showed that TMS significantly improved depressive symptoms in patients with Major Depressive Disorder who have failed antidepressant medication trials.

A major breakthrough in TMS insurance coverage was the decision in January 2011 by the American Medical Association to approve Category 1 CPT codes of 90867 (TMS Motor Threshold Determination), 90868 (TMS treatment), and 90869 (TMS Motor Threshold Redetermination) for TMS treatments. The issuance of these codes demonstrates that TMS therapy has met the AMA's criteria for Category 1 status. Category 1 CPT codes are utilized throughout medicine to bill health plans for medical services. The AMA issues these codes when new technologies and other medical services enter medical practice and are established as an accepted standard of care by the physician specialty performing the service. Furthermore, the American Psychiatric Association included TMS in their 2010 Practice Guidelines as a viable treatment for Major Depressive Disorder.

Over 100 insurance companies have covered TMS upon appeal after an initial rejection. A number of insurance companies recognize the effectiveness of TMS and are offering to cover TMS with prior authorization. NHIC, a Medicare contractor in New England, has adopted a coverage plan for TMS. Our hope is for a groundswell of support to occur throughout the country, so that eventually all insurers will cover TMS therapy for depression.

There is a mounting number of insurers around the country who are developing policies to cover TMS therapy treatment for patients with depression who have not responded to medication therapy. Patients should check with individual insurers for coverage.

Can a denial by the insurance company be appealed?

Neuronetics has contracted with NeuroStar Care Connections (NCC) to initiate prior authorization with insurance companies. Most likely the insurer will turn down the prior authorization, stating that TMS is "investigational" and will recommend ECT, even though ECT is more costly and has many more side effects.

The next step is to file an internal appeal with your insurance company. Subsequently, your TMS provider can help you with the appeal and work with other clinicians to document failed treatment trials and prove that TMS is an appropriate option. In most states insurance companies are mandated to provide two internal appeals in which psychiatrists contracted by the insurance company review the appeal and typically deny TMS treatment.

After going through the two internal appeals, most states have an external appeal process engaging independent psychiatrists from an independent review organization (IPRO) that evaluates the merits of the case. Neuronetics data has shown that there is an increased trend toward success with external appeals when the original denial is reversed and partial or total payment for TMS treatments are paid.

It is important to file the appeals in a timely fashion, as there are deadlines required by the insurance company to successfully file the internal and external appeals. Some states require a filing fee that is reimbursed to you if you win your external appeal.

Treatment rates vary depending on geographic location and out-of-pocket payment may be required. Many TMS practices are offering a variety of payment plans and accept credit cards Flexible Spending Accounts are also a payment option.

Acknowledgements

My heartfelt gratitude goes to the following people:

Joy Patermo who informed me I was writing a book even before I knew I was, and for introducing me to Dr. Randy Pardell.

Randy Pardell for redefining the term, "The Good Doctor". He is an extraordinary physician who refuses to give up on his commitment to his patients. Who, from the outset, has honored and respected my voice in telling this story. And for his enthusiastic support for our shared mission of helping people who suffer with depression. But most of all, for his friendship.

Rosalind Sklar for making my TMS six weeks so enjoyable, and for her continued brilliance in dealing with my insurance company, making sure I have ongoing pre-authorizations for "as needed" TMS treatments.

The doctors and staff at Hartford Hospital for bringing TMS therapy to the Institute of Living and to the folks at Anthem Blue Cross Blue Shield for giving me coverage for TMS. You have all helped save my life.

Susan Emerson MS MSW, for encouraging me to write and for unfailingly supporting my quest for an alternative therapy.

Lisa Tener for being the best book writing coach and editor a new author could ever hope to have, and for her on-going love and support for my writing career. At times she cared as much, if not more, about this book than I was able to muster.

Lisa Tener's *Bring Your Book To Life* class members who were the first to hear my words on paper and kept asking for another chapter. In particular, Anne Burnett, Stacy Corrigan, Nora Hall.

Wilton Writers Workshop: E. Katherine Kerr, Elisabeth Morten, Linda Howard Urbach, all brilliant authors in their own right, for powerful Thursday afternoons where their collective intelligence, compassion, experience, and wisdom provided me with the forum to become a confident and realized writer.

Special thanks to E. Katherine Kerr for her love, support and always knowing when to help me "get present" within the creative process.

Hazel Lazarus for a final proofread and devoted friendship.

(Continued on next page)

Maura Shaw and Joe Tantillo for their initial editing and design contributions.

Steven Robinson for his sensitive photography.

Robert Guy for his cover design expertise..

Lisa Maxwell—a fabulous design coach and teacher. Her willingness to get me through the home stretch will always be remembered.

Members of The TMS Center of the Hudson Valley TMS Support Group for their courage and candor in our monthly meetings.

The doctors, scientists, and staff at Neuronetics for verifying the information in this book to ensure readers are accurately informed about Transcranial Magnetic Stimulation.

Nicholas Pasternack and Miriam Ryan Pasternack for being the extraordinary parents who raised their seven children with style and grace. They've seen it all and love me anyway: Maria Pasternack Hardin, Michael Pasternack, Vincent de Paul Pasternack, Stefan Pasternack, Nicole Pasternack Lalama, Annette Pasternack Lanotte.

Thank you Maria, Michael and Vincent for keeping me honest with the Hartford memories.

Thank you Nicole for believing in this book so passionately and compassionately, and for giving so much of your precious time with editing, cover design, and feedback.

Annetteski for the thoughtful journal, crossword book and art kit to get me through my writer's slumps. The diversions really worked.

And thank you John, Nicholas and Elizabeth Rhodes for your courage in trusting me to write this story.